Oh Why Did I Do That !

... and what to do about it

Revised Edition

Amanda Nicholson

In Acknowledgement Of:

The superb, inspirational writers who have made learning so enjoyable and this publication so necessary,

The wonderful experiences I have had with so-called patients – believe me it was a mutually beneficial encounter,

My friends, colleagues and family.

FOREWORD

Firstly thank you to all who read the first edition of 'Oh Why Did I Do That!? I was amazed at how many people it helped and the positive feedback I received. I feel a bit of a cheat when I receive acclaim for writing a book. As I have said many times, that book simply came out. I was inspired by so many brilliant writers, and also the great research work so many practioners undertake to move our knowledge forward, particularly in the field of mental health. It is one of those areas in which substantial leaps are being taken in very short spaces of time. All areas of science have become involved from radiography to quantum physics. So much work is being done by users of the health services themselves, directing the areas addressed and shaping how treatment evolves. What has also happened is that people as individuals are realizing that what society once saw as a mental health problem, is in reality, a natural part of the human condition, of life. I am personally greatly involved in the promotion of Mindfulness Practice within the NHS. This is an age old ancient wisdom, yet it is one of the most pertinent and successful practices in mental healthcare today. Its foundation is said to have come from the invitation of Buddha himself to 'Come, See'. So simply come; see life as it really is, warts and all the glories. Life may not be perfect but maybe the reason for that is perfect is not a term truly relevant to life.

A year on and with your feedback, I have the opportunity to improve this work, to enable it to be even more useful. There was a call for more relating to Mindfulness Practice, particularly the meditation. That was a task I could not resist. The essence of the book remains the same. It is about coming to know yourself, how you work, why you do the things you do. But included in the title is also '... and what to do about it', and that is where Mindfulness Practice takes the stage. Being Mindful is becoming aware of ourselves in the moment. It sounds hard, but once you start doing it is easy. And the rewards are infinite.

So welcome to the Revised Edition of 'Oh Why Did I Do That!? ... and what to do about it.'

PROLOGUE

This book, whilst being a self-help book, does not entertain the view that either you or your behaviours are flawed; it does not suggest you or your thought processes need fixing.

What it does do is acknowledge that you do what you do for a primarily valid reason; it shows you the rationale behind the way you think and the way you act. The principle is that in imparting that understanding, you become able to appreciate the brilliant working unit that you already are.

For that reason, the aim is not to change you, but add to you. The understanding empowers you to give yourself more options - the ones you want; to gain more control over all that is you, thereby increasing your life possibilities, as you want.

With this new understanding, the internal fights within all of us that exacerbate physical imbalances and sup our energy; depriving us of motivation and making us feel useless, become solved.

To truly appreciate and get the most out of life, you first have to truly appreciate and get the most out of yourself. You have to take that first step. There is no avoidance of that first step ever. There is no short cut, there is no magic carpet. The first step is to appreciate you. When you know how you are working, you will both gain self-appreciation and also you will know how to get the most out of yourself.

As you begin to understand, you will see that you are not wrong, not broken, not flawed. With the self-appreciation that ensues, your mood will lift, your outlook will change and everything about you will heighten and brighten, including your energy levels. From that point, the world is your oyster. Where you go from there, is purely your choice. But as the saying goes 'A journey of a thousand miles must begin with that first step.

This book emerges from a combination of various approaches and philosophies; largely it reflects Mindfulness Principles and explains in real life terms the effects of judgment, acknowledgement and acceptance, and the benefits of being able to live each moment.

It is designed to give genuinely holistic choices. It is written to enable the reader to enhance the quality of their own life.

It acknowledges individuality. No one rule fits all, we are unique and individual.

This book does not seek to take control, but to give it. There are no dos and don'ts, just options.

This book applies to the realities and logistics of our everyday lives. It does not expect the de-motivated individual to suddenly become self-disciplined enough to commence laborious time consuming exercises. It does not expect the already over-run individual to find extra hours each day, in order to cope with their life demands. This is a book that is about real everyday life, every day feelings and every day thoughts.

What I do hope it does is shift how you think, alter your perceptions, thereby altering your responses. But this happens as you begin to know yourself; this happens as you begin to really appreciate just how magnificent you already are.

The aim is that you become the master of you as opposed to the victim of you. The aim is you will know why you did that, whatever that may be. The aim is that next time you will do what is most helpful to you, it may be that again, but at least next time it will be out of choice.

Lastly, reading this book and finding out about you should be fun. Liken this book to taking a walk through a well-stocked clothes store. Try things on; see what fits and what works for you. You decide what you like and what you don't. You can mix and match, and you can choose to wear any or all of these metaphoric clothes or not. My feeling is you will enjoy wearing some of them, some of the time. You will find old favorites, and you will find those you save for special occasions. The point is – that's ok, because the point is - this is about choice. It is totally about what makes you feel good about yourself, because the aim is to show you your best, show you just what you are easily capable of, just what it is you already do that you can make work for you.

The aim is by the end of this book you will have the know-how, the confidence and the desire to exercise your choices about you and your life.

Contents

Our Behavioural Origins – Survival

We do need to start from the beginning, and that beginning is right back to our origins, both as a species and as an individual.

Man has crawled then walked this earth for millennia. Humankind is still here simply because it has survived. Survival is our instinct; we are born hard-wired for survival.

Survival has directed the course of evolution. The whole of the evolutionary process is built upon the need to survive both as an individual and as a species. Successful adaptations that become woven into our genes all link to increased survival ratios.

A seemingly helpless newborn baby has this instinct, this drive; it already has the unlearned know-how to enhance its own chances of survival.

If this little human feels cold, pain, discomfort or hunger, it will cry. Its cry is pitched absolutely perfectly to evoke the mother's instinct.

Mutually interactive maternal/infant instincts ensure the cry of offspring is extremely hard to ignore. Many mothers testify to the fact that when other people's babies cry, it has little effect on them. However, they find it almost impossible to ignore the cry of their own. When baby cries, parents automatically become highly alert.

This is so throughout the animal kingdom. This strategy works, therefore it has survived. It has served us well and we pass this onto our own offspring.

Newborns arrive pre-sensitized and proactive to danger. In humans, the 'Moro' reflex, throwing arms forward and together in a protective position at the sound of a loud noise, quickly develops into the 'startle response' in which the mouth opens, the head lowers and the shoulders and arms sag. Both of these are defensive mechanisms designed to enhance the chances of survival in the presence of danger.

Indeed all animals have their specialist instinctive responses to danger; all are pre-wired to recognise and react to anything that threatens the chance of survival. Danger threatens survival.

This is our origin, this is where we have come from, and this is how we were born into this world as individuals. We still have this instinct to survive. Even as adults, however civilized we think we are, however far we feel we have come, we are still pre-wired to recognise and react to danger, purely because, danger is a threat to our survival.

Soon after birth, human babies begin to imitate facial expressions. There is no understanding of these expressions - that comes later in development. This mimicry is purely 'instinct', the pre-programming that drives the newborn to copy. The effect of this behaviour though is the assured attention of the adult and acceptance into the group. Adult and group attention increases the odds of survival.

As babies become toddlers, this mimicry continues. Their play often copies adults. This is actually so for most mammals and some birds. The youngsters try out life as they perceive it.

Meanwhile, the brain continues to develop, internally incorporating and adopting these behaviours into its brain physiology. It assumes life as it is experiencing it as the norm and makes it the norm. Neural pathways or networks are created and with each use they become strengthened.

Automatic Responses

As the brain grows, and also continuously throughout our life, neural pathways develop. Millions of neurons (nerve cells) create pathways that connect one part of the nervous system to another. Each part of the system used in a particular behaviour becomes networked with the other parts. Movement of limbs, the rate at which the heart and lungs work, sensory information centers (sight, hearing), all become linked enabling them to work together in the blink of an eye to a given cue. We call this cue a trigger.

Neural pathways or networks are always strengthened through use. Each time a behaviour or response is used, neurons grow more tendrils, making that pathway faster and more effective in its role of receiving and sending signals quickly. Each part of the nervous system 'contacted' performs a necessary function toward the outcome of the behaviour enlisted. Neural pathways direct these actions and reactions. The stronger a neural pathway, the less conscious of it we are.

We can recognise these strong neural pathways as habits or automatic responses, things we do without conscious thought.

To understand this process, let's use the example of learning to drive.

When we initially start learning to drive we are conscious of every movement we have to make; one foot on clutch, the other on accelerator, carefully bringing one foot up as the other goes down; hands on steering wheel, changing gear and indicating; looking forwards and glancing backwards through mirrors. At first we wonder how we will ever be able to accomplish all these different tasks at the same time and whilst moving! However, as we practice, it becomes easier, and eventually, driving – doing this combination of tasks at once, becomes second nature, habit; we don't think about it anymore. This behaviour – 'driving' goes subconscious. It becomes automatic.

It may surprise you to hear 'driving' referred to as behaviour but it is just that. The definition of behaviour is – ' *v. a reaction, or combination of actions and reactions.*' Driving is an example of behaviour and it will help if we begin to think of all behaviours in this same way, namely, a set of actions and reactions.

The way in which we act or react, the way in which we 'behave' in varying situations is what we do. Whether behaviours are consciously or subconsciously driven, they are simply a set of actions and reactions. They can be altered. There is always potential for choice. The aim of this book is to show you that choice. It is not written to make that choice for you; it is designed to give you the options.

Once a reaction or combination of reactions goes subconscious, our conscious mind becomes free to learn or think about something else.

Interestingly, no judgment, no label of wrong or right affects the growth or strength of neural pathways. The process is not affected by whether or not the behaviour is moral or strategically beneficial. The subconscious readily automates any behaviour that is persistently used. It is use that causes these neural pathways to strengthen. With use the neurons physically grow more tendrils and consequently these various behaviours become automatic. Cue - key in ignition, sound of engine, we 'drive', all those different actions and reactions carried out in split seconds. We carry on acting and reacting to the road signals around us using our automatic pilot. We literally don't consciously think about it anymore.

Isn't that amazing? When you stop and think about it, you have to agree that driving is an amazing feat of the mind.

The same process applies to learning to play an instrument, learning a second language, learning grammar, how to count, how to multiply and detract. Everything you put your mind to and do consistently, eventually goes subconscious and becomes automatic. This applies to any continuously used behaviour in any realm of life. We carry out thousands upon thousands of automatic behaviours every day. Your mind is a magnificent tool. Do you truly appreciate just what it is doing each and every second of each and every day?

Now cast your mind back to that baby. It came into this world consciously knowing nothing but having an instinct to survive. It learnt to walk, talk, use a toilet, indeed to control its own bladder. It learnt how to chew, how to interact, how to move, how to balance. That baby is you. Millions upon millions of neural pathways, continuously strengthening through use, all 'happening' without you ever having to give them a conscious thought. Millions of neural pathways are literally directing your behaviour without your conscious knowledge.

As we grow, as we gain more experience and more knowledge, we learn alternatives. As adults we have many alternatives as to how we behave in various situations. However, it is the strongest neural pathway that will always take precedence if left unchecked.

It is a simple case of circuitry; the impulses take the easiest, fastest, most used route, the line of least resistance. The more we display a particular behaviour to a given cue, the more likely that behaviour will be the default reaction to that particular trigger.

Our origins, our genetic predispositions, our own individual life experience have all thus far dictated the strength of the neural pathways that direct our current behaviours.

However, we are adaptive. It is adaptation capability that made them grow strong in the first place. We still have that adaptive ability. These neural pathways are changeable. This is called brain plasticity.

Brain plasticity is the brain's ability to change, to reroute. Much research has been done in the area of brain plasticity, and it has been proven beyond doubt that different areas of the brain can take over different areas of responsibility.

When a pathway or network is not used, the tendrils of the neurons involved wither away. That pathway becomes less strong and as such loses its place in the ranking of default use.

If we want choice, we simply bring automatic behaviours back to the attention of our conscious and begin to do things in a different way. Whilst first time we do this it feels strange and it so easy, each time we do it becomes easier. Remember growth is promoted by use. Decline is promoted by non-use. The more we use an automatic response, the stronger it grows. The more we halt it, the faster it shrinks. It is that simple.

The Fight/Flight Response

Though many things affect behaviour, survival remains one of the primary concerns of our nervous system. We mentioned the 'startle response' and 'Moro-reflex' in babies; in larger children and adults, in the presence of perceived danger, this is superseded by what we call the fight/flight response.

Sometimes, a certain trigger, a particular circumstance will evoke your fight/flight response; you will experience fear. This experience will cause the blood vessels supplying oxygen and nutrients to many organs in your torso, such as your digestive system, to constrict; but the vessels supplying your muscles and your brain will expand. Your lungs will begin to take in more oxygen; you will breathe faster and more deeply. Your heart will beat faster to deliver this oxygenated blood more rapidly to the areas of your body that will enable you to run or fight. Your pupils will dilate. Even your immune system will be activated, giving immediate protection from infection of potential wounds caused by teeth, claws, etc. You will feel highly alert and ready to act.

These physiological responses are caused by the release of adrenaline, cortisol, noradrenalin and epinephrine. These hormones are activated by the release of adrenocorticotropic hormone (ACTH) from the pituitary gland. The release of ACTH is triggered by corticotrophin-releasing hormone from the hypothalamus.

The big words don't matter; you do all this in response to something that frightens you. You didn't have to have prior knowledge of these long names or this process, you didn't have to know anything about it; you do all this anyway. You have been able to carry out this process since the day you were born.

This fight/flight response is controlled by your autonomic nervous system. In normal circumstance, you have no conscious control over it. You do not need to have conscious control over it, indeed it would not be effective to have.

If a hungry lion walked into the room at this moment and you began consciously wondering about the situation, i.e. is it really a lion? Is it really hungry? When did it last eat? What shall I do? Trust me; you will be eaten before you have the time to ponder the first two questions.

The fact that we have no conscious control over the autonomic nervous system aids our survival. We run before we have had time to think about it. And moreover, our body has become highly prepared to run or fight before we have even consciously recognised the situation as being what it is.

The autonomic nervous system constitutes the pre-hard wiring, the pre-existing neural networks we spoke about at the beginning of this book. It keeps you safe; it enables you to stay alive. It is responsible for keeping you breathing and keeping your heart beating; and it is responsible for this fight/flight response.

The above mentioned processes occur in split seconds. Acknowledge you are wonderful just the way you are in this respect. Don't change it, don't fix it, it works perfectly.

However, we often experience this fight/flight response in situations that do not actually threaten our survival.

Someone we don't like may walk into the room. He/she is not a hungry lion and doesn't actually threaten our survival, but they may still evoke the fight/flight response in us. We may watch something on the television that is disturbing, and whilst it may be highly unpleasant, it is only on the TV and it does not threaten our survival. However, it may still provoke that fight/flight response. We may become concerned about something we have done or not done at work or in some other area of life. Again, even though it is not directly life threatening, we experience this fight/flight response.

Because the fight/flight response occurs to stimulus that frightens us, it responds to our feeling fear, it may be set in action by anything that makes us fearful.

In our modern day life many things frighten us but don't immediately threaten our survival. Not being able to pay our bills may frighten us. Not doing well at work may frighten us. Worrying we or our children may not pass an exam may frighten us and them. Many things act as triggers for the fight/flight response that do not immediately threaten our survival.

When this happens, if left unchecked, we suffer symptoms of stress.

In appropriate circumstances, when we have successfully run out of the way of the hungry lion, when we have utilised those strengthened legs and our hearts and lungs have done their bit, our parasympathetic nervous system reverses the process caused by those hormones and returns our systems to 'normal mode'.

However, when we don't carry out the fight or flight process, i.e. when we don't either run or fight, the cues to our parasympathetic nervous system are not activated. Our body and mind stay heightened, alert, prepared to fight or run. If this state continues for longer than it should; our systems become stressed.

Prolonged or continuous, unnecessary fight/flight responses have very unhelpful effects on us physically and psychologically. In mental health we call this condition Anxiety.

The potential physical effects of stress and anxiety include damage to our immune systems, headaches, muscle pain, insomnia, fatigue, upset stomach, to name but a few. There are disturbances in our behaviours. We may become easily angry or irritable, restless, experience lack of concentration, lack of motivation and even become depressed. We find it hard to sleep; we don't perform normal tasks effectively. There are physiological scientific reasons for all these symptoms, it does make sense.

And meantime, our systems are working as they should; the primary reason for our response was we perceived danger. Our bodies and minds have done nothing wrong, they are protecting us. We simply got frightened by the wrong thing. That particular response to that particular trigger may not have been necessary, and it did not prove helpful.

So we need to learn how to help ourselves stay well and healthy. We need to know how to engage our own cognitive abilities.

So what can we do? Firstly, identify when you are experiencing the fight/flight response. This is not hard, you will know. You will feel fear or anger; a tightening of your stomach, your heart beating faster and deepening of your breaths. In the absence of a hungry lion or other factor that may be an immediate threat to your survival, endeavor to establish what is causing this reaction.

Sometimes you may not be able to pinpoint exactly why you are feeling this way, but you will be able to identify something. Don't judge it. Don't say it cannot be that as that is not something I should be fearful of. Allow yourself to acknowledge what is triggering this response without fear of judgment. At this point you don't have to tell anyone if you don't want to, but acknowledge it to yourself and know without doubt that this is happening for valid reason, even if you do not know what this reason is right now. Something is causing you to feel fear. Give your own system credit for having made that response automatic as it is reacting to save your life. Know that for this response to have become automatic to that given cue, there was at some point a valid reason why it made you fearful. Remember you weren't always this big and this able; that response may have been enlisted when you were smaller. It doesn't matter what or why, it matters that you give your own system credibility for having this reaction. It takes only split seconds to acknowledge this to yourself.

Next acknowledge you are in a high state of arousal and do something that will help your system to naturally eliminate the physical changes that have occurred in you. Do something physical. Pace up and down awhile, go run up a flight of stairs, take a brisk walk around the garden, jump up and down on the spot, but do something physical. This will assist your parasympathetic nervous system to release the hormones that bring your physiology back into normal mode. We call this homeostasis, the ability our bodies naturally have to regulate our own physiology and keep in it balance. Acknowledge you have this capability also. Acknowledge just how clever and amazing you already are. If you can help your parasympathetic nervous system out by running a lap or two, do it. If you can do something bigger or better at this precise moment, do so, but very often you won't be in the right circumstances. So do what you can, make your body physically work hard for at least a moment or two and your body will do the rest for you. Allow your system to see the job through. It has been designed to work perfectly, so allow it. Don't fight it; don't beat yourself up for feeling fear as this will exacerbate your fear. Acknowledge what is happening, acknowledge how clever it is and work with it. Whilst you are doing this, engage your own cognitive abilities. Think about where you are right now. Assure yourself that nothing is immediately threatening your survival. Acknowledge this is a worry, not a threat on your life.

If you are in a situation where some physical activity is not feasible right away, then carry out an exercise I call Square Breathing. It takes a maximum of twenty seconds and is enough to halt any inappropriate automatic behavioral response to the arousal you are feeling, particularly the alternative to running, which is fight.

For example, someone may have said something to you that has elicited this fight/flight response. It may be an automated reaction to punch them or carry out some other behaviour that is in line with the fight response. It is likely this will be an inappropriate response, and not be effective in bringing about any desired outcome, even though you may feel the urge and it may make you feel better for that instant.

Square breathing consists of breathing in to the count of 5 and mentally drawing the first line of a square whilst doing so. Then breathe out to the count of 5 mentally drawing the second line of the square. Breathe in again to the count of 5, mentally drawing the third line of the square and out again to the count of 5, mentally completing the square.

This has the effect of slowing down your breathing and also bringing your automatic physiological responses to the attention of the cognitive areas of your brain. Remember that these cognitive areas had been bypassed so you don't start pondering the hungry lion. This breathing exercise as well as calming your physical system, helps you to bring the whole situation to the attention of your conscious, enabling you to realise the actual lack of clear and present danger in this precise moment.

This exercise is enough to bring the situation back into some sort of conscious control. You will calm somewhat, though you may still feel aroused.

However, you will have given yourself the ability to begin to think consciously and relatively calmly. Importantly, it halts the automatic response long enough to stop you from thumping the person in front of you and regretting it the minute you do so. It works on the same principle as the old saying, 'take a deep breath and count to 10'.

My next recommendation is to remove yourself from the situation, maybe tell the person you are not prepared to discuss this at this time. However you do it, just remove yourself if you can, even if just for a while. Once removed, you have more time to address the physical reactions that have occurred in your body as well as time to put the whole situation into another perspective, which we will talk about later.

Sometimes just the mere thought of something produces this fight/flight response. Again, acknowledge what you are feeling and acknowledge it is valid to feel this way. However, also acknowledge that you are not going to be able to effectively address why you are feeling this way when in this heightened state of arousal. Acknowledge your system has disengaged your cognitive (conscious) processes and that you are in fight/flight mode. Do something physical if you can even if it is just a pace up and down. Promise yourself you will come back to it if the current circumstances don't allow for calm reflection at this time.

The most effective time to come back to the subject of what instigated the fight/flight response in you is when you are feeling calm, safe and secure. This may be when you are alone in your room, or maybe when you are talking with your therapist or best friend. That is the time to reflect on whatever triggered this response. That is the time to plan alternative responses should it happen again. It may be helpful to you to explore why this particular thing triggers that response, particularly if it has become a phobia, but this is not always necessary and indeed not always helpful. Regurgitating old fears, trying to sort out the past, doesn't always help. We cannot undo the past; we cannot keep hold of it. Sometimes it is not helpful to keep going over old events.

Esther Hicks explained this principle well during a seminar promoting her book 'The Astonishing Power of Emotions'. She spoke of a journey she undertook, totally reliant on her satellite navigation system for directions. Some way into the journey, the satnav informed her she was going the wrong way and directed her to turn around. She felt sure she had followed the instructions to this point. This perplexed her and she suggested to her husband that they go back to where they were, retrace their journey and find out where they went wrong. Her husband replied, 'Why don't we just keep going the right way from here'.

It is not always necessary to know why or where something went wrong, just acknowledge it did and carry on the right way from the point you are at now.

We are all at the point we are now at. Whatever has happened in the past, whatever we feel went wrong, we are here now. Here is the point to go forward from. Often there is no need to retrace our steps.

There is always a point though to choosing our next step and ensuring it is one we want to take, not one that we will frustratingly ask 'Oh Why Did I Do That?' about.

Mindfulness practice is about living in This Moment. It is always helpful to do so. There are so many things about this moment that we miss. Our experience of life is moment by moment. If we recreate the tragedies of the past in our own minds now, we 'feel' that experience now and actually miss this moment of life as it is now.

Personality and the Introduction of Judgment

Many different things influence the formation of behaviours. It is always easy to think of traumatic life events and instinct for survival, but these are not the only things that influence our actions and reactions. Life is about more than hunting for the next meal and avoiding the next predator. Life has become more intricate. Behaviours have become about more than immediate survival.

Our behaviors affect the way we feel internally. They affect how others perceive us, and consequently how they in turn react to us, how they behave, and importantly how they perceive us.

All of our different behaviours, all the various sets of actions and reactions we utilize to given cues, are summed up by others as our 'personality'. Common factors about our different behaviours are labeled and referred to as our personality type. Very often, some of the characteristics of just one of our common behaviours attracts a personality label.

Think about some famous people you know, actors, sportsmen, how would you describe their personality? The way they behave on just one public interview may be enough for us to feel sufficiently informed to describe their personality. The way they behave during one sporting competition may be enough for us to deliver a personality judgment about their personality. We often refer to people who are in the media as 'famous personalities'.

Our western culture just loves labels, and labels carry judgments. We each hold perceptions regarding these various personality labels, and very often these are preconceptions. This is woven intrinsically throughout our everyday life and becomes apparent in our use of language.

Judgment is evoked by language and how we use it to communicate. It may not be overt, obvious, but it is very powerful and influential on our daily life, and therefore on our behaviours. Cultural and peer judgment have a big influence on our actions and reactions.

If I were to ask 'What personality are you?', it would not be unusual for you to react defensively to that question as your instinct, that neural activity in response to given cues, will warn you a judgment of you will be formatted on your reply.

If I asked someone else that same question about you in front of you, your ears are very likely to hang on every word of their answer. You may even notice you have become highly prepared to react, alert. Be it to agree with their comments or disagree, you may well become physically aroused to react, to behave in response to my words. Language and how it is used has a profound effect on our behaviours.

Furthermore, cultural and social conditioning has taught us the inferences of words alongside their actual meanings. The words 'behaviour' and 'personality' are both strong examples of this. As children we are taught to 'behave ourselves'. Classic comedy series satirically amuse us with our male counterparts 'behaving' badly, however fondly. 'To 'behave' is often translated as to 'be good' or to 'do the right thing'. This is despite the fact that behaviour literally means a set of actions and reactions, and consequently, we are in reality, 'behaving' all of the time.

Our society decrees that various sets of persistently used behaviours define our personality, and the inference that comes with the word personality is extremely personal; the inference is, it defines you. When someone describes our personality, they are generally talking about our common or well-known behaviour, yet that description is accepted as who we are. A lady who gives many sets of instructions is labeled 'bossy'; a man who walks away from fights rather than get involved in them may attract the label of 'weak' or 'spineless'. A sportsman may be labeled 'aggressive'. A child who gets good grades may be referred to as 'clever' or even as 'nerdy'. The label is not merely attached to the particular behaviour they utilised at a specific time, it becomes, incorrectly in my opinion, attributed directly AS the person.

We also use language in this way when referring to certain medical diagnoses. For example we often say 'she is diabetic' as opposed to 'she suffers from diabetes'. Or we say 'he is epileptic' as opposed to 'he suffers from epilepsy'. Interestingly though we do not do this with all diagnoses, we do not label people in this way that are suffering from influenza, the common cold or cancer. In those cases we refer to that person as having the disease or condition rather than referring to them as the disease or condition.

These are strong linguistic influences. They cause a reaction.

Along with most personality labels comes an inference of good or bad. Though not directly said, it is implied. The general implication behind bossy or weak is not good. The general implication is that bossy and weak are not sought after personality traits. We tend not to want to be called bossy or weak. The inference behind clever is good. We quite like it when we are referred to as clever.

The way in which we speak our language can also alter the inference. The tone of our voice and the inflections and punctuation we apply, can alter the meaning. If we say in a derisive tone 'oh how clever' with the intent of putting someone down, 'clever' as a personality trait takes on a different meaning and becomes not so desirable.

The main point though is we live our lives labeling people as behaviours. Due to the way we both speak and interpret the spoken word, these personality labels become people labels.

We all 'feel' the inferences, both in what we speak out and what we hear in. We 'feel' the implication; we become aware of the judgment in terms of good or bad. Our cultural use of language is very judgmental and therefore very influential over our behaviours.

By nature we are attuned to avoid 'bad'. It provokes a negative response and we shy away from it; it 'feels' similar or in some way linked to danger. It has a negative effect on our experience.

It is necessary to become aware of good/bad judgments. It is good to become aware of these judgmental implications both when we speak and when we are spoken to.

Again, the 'what' to do about it becomes, pay attention to this moment. Notice and acknowledge just what you are inferring when you speak. Become aware of what you are really trying to say, even though you may not be able or willing to say directly. Think about your reasons for doing this and acknowledge these to yourself, also without judgment. If you felt compelled to speak in a certain way, ask yourself why. Reflect on what did you 'feel'? At what point was that feeling felt? What made you feel that way?

You begin to see that what you 'feel' is also as influential on your behaviour, your subsequent actions and reactions, as what actually occurred.

And that's OK. It's there for a reason. For the time being go with it, don't judge it. The reason I say this is because when considering judgment, even in terms of beneficial and non-beneficial, there are nearly always elements of both.

One of the principles of Mindfulness is Non-Judgment. Living in the moment is about accepting what is in this moment as 'what exists'. Change occurs from this stable point into the next moment. Now is as now is - there is no point to judgment. It 'is' anyway. And no stable change can occur from a point of what isn't.

Socially Accepted Behaviors

Continuing the story of our baby, survival instinct has programmed this helpless bundle of life to know that being near its parents, particularly mother will increase its chances of survival.

Being nursed by mum equates to a uniquely prepared nourishing food supply on demand. The interactive instincts are so powerful that the cry of baby may cause the mother to lactate. Initially this tailor made food supply protects baby from unseen dangers, such as bacteria and viruses. During the first few days of the baby's life, the mother is able to share her immune system with her offspring. It is highly likely the mother has developed immunity to many things normally present in her own environment. This is now baby's environment, so this immunity is precisely effective.

Being physically held by parents also means warmth, i.e. protection from temperatures that threaten survival. This same cuddle also provides veritable protection from predators. A potential predator that would lunch on a lone baby is highly likely to think twice about attempting to attack something ten times larger first, in order to get to it.

Hence these preconditioned behaviours, 'baby cries, parents pick up, baby stops crying' or 'toddler wakes in the night, finds mummy's bed, goes back to sleep, (albeit dislodging daddy in the process)', are highly honed and very successful strategies for increasing the odds of survival.

Some of us may already have tut-tutted in disapproval at the mention of toddler getting into mummy's bed. Although we are discussing instinctive behaviours driven by very logical drives for the purpose of survival, we have also learned our society's opinion of acceptable behaviour. In the West, we discourage these infantile behaviours very early. (Just remember that term – infantile behaviour, I will come back to it in a minute.)

We live in houses, generally with more than one bedroom. We deem baby should sleep in its own room; if not a separate room, then definitely a separate cot. We know, and if we don't the professionals will tell us, when baby cries do not keep picking it up; when toddler climbs into your bed, put it back in its own bed. We teach our young from the earliest age that pure instinct will not pay off. We are attempting to teach our very young how to behave as deemed right by our culture, our way of life. These are called learned behaviours.

The level of compliance with these learned behaviors often attract a high degree of judgment using a scale measuring right at one end and wrong at the other. A child that keeps getting into mum's bed at night is often referred to as being naughty. A child that sleeps quietly all through the night in its own room is good. In terms of instinctive survival behaviour, the latter child isn't good. In the jungle or the forest, it would most likely not survive, but when judged in terms of acceptable social behaviour it becomes the good one.

Put simply, we judge these behaviours in accordance with perceived levels of social acceptance. That becomes our judgmental ruler; we give no thought to the origin of the behaviour.

Now back to the term infantile behaviour – what feelings of judgment did that stir in you? It is even used as a derogatory phrase applied to adults. How many infantile behaviours can you think of and then easily categorise into terms of good and bad, or right and wrong?

Now define in what way these behaviours are right and in what way are they wrong. Try to think of some circumstance in which that behaviour may have been effective or helpful. Remember who our subject is, namely a tiny helpless infant. Think of its abilities versus its needs. What I am asking you to do here is use a different ruler; I am asking you to measure using a different judgmental scale. This will cause you to view the same thing from a different perspective.

Now try to do this exercise for each behaviour you thought of from the opposite side, from the other person's point of view. For example, think how this behaviour is perceived by mums and dads who know that baby will be fed every four hours and don't even consider the possibility of predators in this part of town. Think about what the Health Visitor might say to the parents when advising about these behaviours. What would Grandma say?

Now think in terms of an adult utilizing these infantile behaviors? Would these behaviours be seen as problem behaviors or do we start to understand their purpose? Be honest. Don't judge your answers. Do things change when seeing them from a different position, a different perspective?

Again Mindfulness Practice develops our use of varying perspectives. Our minds have the capability of understanding many perspectives, and our perspectives highly influence our experience of life. More on this later.

Now going back to our exercise, when you were thinking of whether behaviors were good or bad, did you momentarily hesitate over being honest? For one split second did you question whether your opinion was in line with the current generally held opinion? If you are doing this exercise with someone else, did you wonder what they would think of your judgments?

How often do current opinions with regard to how we should deal with our young change? Should we put them to sleep on their backs, their fronts or their sides? Who knows what we will be advised to do this year.

The point is that current opinion often changes, yet it is common for us to expect ourselves to be continuously abreast of it. This is basically due to the fact that we fear external judgment. Hence often before we say something, we hesitate, grasping for cues to decipher if we are in line with current opinion. If we don't, we often end up thinking 'Oh I wish I hadn't said that!'

In other areas of life do you do this? Do you ever think something is so but hesitate to say it in case others don't agree, or alternatively realise after that it wasn't currently held opinion and beat yourself up for saying it? This is self-judgment.

Self- Judgment

Recognise that self-judgment is an automatic behaviour also. Our instant reaction to measure ourselves along a scale of right to wrong, judging, is a behaviour we have also learned to do and do incredibly often. We do not merely judge externally, we automatically are continuously judging ourselves. We do not try to judge, we do it automatically. We measure normal, abnormal, usual, unusual, right and wrong, acceptable and unacceptable nearly all of the time. Our language evokes it. Our culture evokes it. Judgment is so often called upon that it has gone subconscious also.

Now we begin to realise just what is involved in the formation of our habitual behaviours. Also now we can begin to understand the reality of and understand the presence of our common feeling of internal dissent, that inner battle, that feeling of unease we are often feeling.

We now begin to realise that we all have conflicting directions and instructions emanating from our own subconscious. We have conflicting drivers calling for different behaviours. We have conflicting automatic responses all bustling to be the first to affect their reaction to given cues. No wonder we end up asking 'Oh Why Did I Do that?'

As previously stated, very often the strongest neural pathway wins. It will work the quickest. The neurons have grown many tendrils for the impulse to travel through. It is the least line of resistance. The consequence of this automatic response is measured by how often we say or think, 'I wish I hadn't done that'. The common and actual answer to our question 'Oh, Why Did I Do That!?' is very simply - that particular neural network fired the quickest.

This internal fight is a major factor in chronic depression and anxiety. We are often acting and reacting in a way we wish we hadn't. We are also subconsciously striving to do right by more than one set of rules; often unable to evaluate which set of rules we should play by in each different circumstance.

Now we begin to realize why life sometimes feels so hard. So often there is this direct internal conflict between our natural instincts, our desires and our learned socially acceptable' behaviours.

Simplistically Freud referred to the Id - the bit of us responding with instinctive behaviours and the Ego as the bit of us responding with learned behaviours. Freud felt many behavioral and mental disorders were due to this conflict between the two. Constantly society and culture demand sets of behaviours far removed from our basic instincts. Our baser drives become suppressed very often, minimally giving us a feeling of discomfort and unease, and at the other extreme, causing physical and physiological problems.

As shown brilliantly by Sir Robert Winston in his TV series and book, 'Human Instinct', many of the behaviours we think of as not acceptable in our culture, have a basis in instinctive behaviour for very survival valid reasons. Many of the things we experience and react to in a way we later question, become very understandable when we are aware of the original source of the reaction.

Jealousy is a prime example of this. Next time you feel jealous, don't beat yourself up. Rather understand that jealousy is an inherent response to protect the continuation of our own genes. It is the equivalent of our DNA's fight/flight response. No prehistoric man wanted to nurture someone else's genes, he would have considered that an extortionate waste of his resources. Actually he probably wouldn't have considered it at all, rather just gone along with his own instinctual reaction.

However society now shows disdain for emotions like jealousy, thinking them uncivilized. We do at some point or another though all feel jealousy. It is worth thinking about why before we join forces with society and beat ourselves up.

Recognise your behaviour for what it was originally intended for before you label yourself as bad. Being honest with yourself goes two ways. It is not just about identifying what is wrong with us. It is also about acknowledging our own valid bases. When seen in the right perspective, or when measured by the appropriate measuring tool, we begin to see what is right with us. Behaviours we may initially think we do not want to own become seen under both lights, or even under all lights. We realize that in the right circumstances, this automatic behaviour, this habit of ours, may prove helpful. We may decide that if we ever are in the presence of a predator or a threat, or even a major catastrophe, then this behaviour is not only the most appropriate one but our actual survival may depend on it.

Do not automatically resort to assuming that behaviours are good or bad. Use the measure of effective or not effective relevant to the particular set of circumstances you are using them in. The more behaviours you have at your disposal, the wider your choice.

This is about choice and I reiterate - the choice is yours. I merely want to open your mind and impart enough knowledge for you to make informed choices about yourself and your own life, about yourself and your own behaviours.

My aim is that by the end of this book you can recognise your own automatic behaviours, evaluate their effectiveness in a particular set of circumstances and make an informed choice at the required moment. You may decide to keep behaviours, modify them or oust them completely, but it becomes your own choice, and using the principles and practices of Mindfulness, you become able to make numerous informed, creative and unique choices, as you release the vast libraries of your subconscious into your own choice mix.

As an aid to understanding this concept further, think of owning a toolbox. Imagine in your toolbox you have a state of the art hammer. This hammer provides you with excellent grip, its light weight enables you to use it easily and with applied direction, and the head delivers a forceful blow. Any situation that requires a hammer, use it, this thing hammers! It truly is an exceptional hammer. Imagine your instinctive behaviours to be this hammer.

However, should your desired outcome be to remove a tiny screw from an expensive watch so you can replace the battery, your hammer, however excellent, is not the most effective tool for the job. A tiny screwdriver, ineffective for many other jobs, becomes the ideal choice.

It is the same with our behaviours, in one instance, one set of behaviours will be most applicable, most effective and in another the same set of behaviours may be totally catastrophic, metaphorically smashing the beautiful timepiece we so wanted to carry on wearing. Applying a set of behaviours that does not assist in achieving the desired end result, is simply self-sabotage. Self-sabotage is rarely what we intend to do, but is so often what we do 'do'.

Meditation enables us to quiet the constant habitual chatter our cognitive minds impose upon our daily existence. Those jabbering thoughts we all have most of every day are the pre-recordings we live by again and again. These lead to the same perspectives of essentially different circumstances day in and day out. They are full of prejudices and expectations and literally shape our daily experience of life. Our minds are actually vast arenas in which we have the ability to create new, unique, forever changing perspectives, and to view life differently moment by moment. This process actually creates our experience of life. We experience life as we are thinking it, rather than life as we could truly see it. Visapanna or Insight Meditation gives us the ability to hush that incessant droning chatter that is our conscious thought. It enables us to see each moment in a different way and it gives us access to the vast array of responses that are really at our disposal, that are actually already in our toolbox. And of course, experience and knowledge give us both more tools and unique combinations of tools for different situations and circumstances.

We don't have to keep repeating the same self-sabotaging responses.

Self-Esteem, Self-Perception and Self-Awareness

These acts or behaviours that become self-sabotaging lead to feelings of low self- esteem. We emotionally beat ourselves up, pull our own hair and question why we did that. We begin to think of ourselves as useless as we fall victim to our own responses. We automatically judge ourselves negatively.

Low self-esteem is a common factor in the diagnosis of depression and anxiety related disorders. Apart from being a symptom of depression and anxiety, low self- esteem is also thought to be a contributing factor to these disorders, a cause. Healthy levels of self-esteem are referred to as a protective factor against such disorders developing and also remedial when they do already exist.

It is therefore important to understand what self-esteem is, how it is recognised, how it is gained and how it affects our own wellbeing. It is also important that we understand the difference between self-esteem, self-perception and self- awareness. For that we can return to our exploration of our baby's development.

Research shows that babies do not hold a sense of separate self. This sense of individual self begins to develop and emerge around the age of two.

We do however identify from birth, the effect of an act or behaviour. We learn 'I cry - mummy feeds me' or 'I cry – mummy picks me up', or the opposite if so, and we learn that very quickly and easily. Although initially powered by an instinctive drive, we become very aware of the effects of our behaviors from day one. At this point the awareness is merely of the behaviour (cause) combined with environmental or social reaction (effect). A behaviour that gets a desired outcome will be kept, used and therefore that neural pathway will become strengthened. Babies and young children operate in this mode of cause and effect, powered by the drive to increase chances of survival. They do not hold a sense of moral right and wrong. They do not possess judgment as we know it.

From around the age of two, children become able to compare and categorise themselves against others in terms of age, gender and size. This self-awareness, i.e. awareness of what they did, (behaviour), begins to develop into self-perception. They then begin to think in terms of comparison, i.e. 'I see myself as shorter than him' or 'Her hair is longer than mine'.

However they are still only measuring, or judging in terms of fact. All the time 'he is bigger than me' or 'her hair is longer than mine' has no detrimental effect as perceived by the drive for survival, they won't have a problem with it.

However, the minute that child perceives the girl with the long hair is getting all the adult attention, or the boy who is bigger just knocked her over; the other does become perceived as a potential threat to survival. The young child, our subject, will react instinctively. The child may pull the long hair of the girl, or cry vehemently when knocked over by the boy, even if not hurt.

However at this point, the young child comes into contact with judgment measured by right and wrong; he/she gets told off, scolded!

Jumping into the mind of that child, and using my two year old measuring judgment of effective and non-effective, if I were able to verbalize the offending event, I may narrate something much like this: " I pulled the girls hair, I attacked her to make her go away in order to retrieve the adult attention back to me. Her pretty hair was causing her to have all the adult attention. Hey, if some predator comes now, this is not good, they could have me for lunch and nobody would notice. My survival requires I get adult attention, so I need to be rid of her. My instinctive drive is to attack. I will either pull off that long hair or I will make her run away."

However, the outcome I achieved was not effective. Carrying on the child's version of events - "...but my instinctive behaviour has caused my protectors, the adults to be angry or cross with me. Now my perceived protectors are acting as if they are a threat to me. Now they have attributed a label called jealousy to me because I pulled that girl's hair."

Now as an infant I don't know what jealousy is, but I do know I have not achieved a reaction that was helpful to me. However the girl who takes all the attention of the adults is still perceived as a threat to my survival. I am still experiencing fear. I don't like her.

At this point, I am still reacting only in terms of the most effective means of survival. Now, though my survival is still being threatened, so I begin to learn about judgment in terms of social right and wrong, and begin to incorporate this right/wrong judgment with effective and non-effective, because if I gain the wrath of the big ones in my social group, my survival is severely threatened. Therefore the adults' perception of right and wrong has now become important to me. I still do not understand why my behaviour was wrong. I have no knowledge of good and bad, I am thus far merely pre-programmed to survive. However, belonging to a pack is survival. I cannot make it on my own, so I adapt, I learn behaviors. Mummy tells me to be nice and play with the girl, so even though I don't like her, with hackles up I play with her.

This is the point we come into contact with social judgment, but we do not yet understand it. However, it so severely threatens our own perceived chance of survival, we do not question it. We accept it. Be it morally right, logically right or not, we learn not to question the opinion of the many. We accept by default, because to not accept poses a threat to survival.

We now begin to understand why we care about the opinions of the many. We now see that in reality we do care what people think. It is our nature, it is part of our basic make-up, our pre-programming, and we need to care because we need to operate as part of a pack. Isolation is not conducive to survival.

As adults, are we are still caught in that stage in one sense or another? As adults, how many societal rights and wrongs do we accept without question, purely because the instinct to maintain the protection of our social group is so strong?

But is our current perception correct? Is our survival really so compromised if we question?

On reflection, we may find that it is not. When we bring our attention to the moment on purpose, we may find we are still just behaving in a purely automated way. Our social group will not necessarily turn predator if we make another choice. In reality, we do have the ability to make choices based on desires and wishes. Life is not just about survival at this point.

Let's carry on through our own development.

By puberty this sense of self, this self-awareness in comparison to others incorporates areas such as beliefs and behaviours. At this point, we are still developing both self-perception and self-awareness, by evaluating the effect of self and of self-action on our environment and as part of our social group. Consequently, we may even decide to grow our own hair! On the whole, teenagers are big on fashion, it is important to them. It identifies them with a peer group.

Along with these self-perceptions we commence self-judgment, influenced by the opinions of family, friends and generalized society viewpoints.

We are also developing our own rule of judgment; we are developing our own measuring tool with which we judge ourselves and others by. Any element of self-perception that appears to attract a judgment of acceptable or unacceptable, right or wrong will affect not only our adolescent self-perception, but also the development of that adolescent measuring tool.

It is really important for us to realise at this point that each individual's measuring tool is uniquely individual. Please write this down, or mark this page, because this is of major relevance and we do come back to it later.

For now though we are investigating self-esteem.

Social judgment often comes in terms of academic achievements, financial or material standing, physical attributes and both internal and external judgments of personality based on behaviours (actions and reactions).

Confusion arises when unexpected judgments or reactions are caused by a particular behaviour, achievement or attribute. If understanding is not reached, self-esteem then becomes affected.

So-called self-sabotaging behaviours are both a cause of and a product of self-criticism, a negative sense of self, i.e. low self-esteem. This is how it works.

We initially behaved in a way that came naturally to us, simply because it was a strong automatic reaction to a given cue. At that moment there was no wrong or right, it just was. However, when it did not achieve the desired result, not only do we receive judgment from others, we begin to measure our self with our own judgmental measuring tool of good and bad. We technically began to judge ourselves as bad or stupid, turn against our self, even though we may not understand why it was unsuccessful. Our own developing automatic judging system turns inward.

This is what we call low self-esteem, and when viewed in this light, it is easy to see why it is so self-destructive. It is also easy to see how this becomes a recurrent negative cycle.

The initial ineffective behaviour is judged as bad, without clear understanding of what bad really is. Therefore, any replacement behaviour is merely a stab in the dark. We falter; we have a drive to protect ourselves, but we internally perceive this as 'bad, not done, but don't know why'. We therefore automatically begin to protect ourselves from our own judgment, and often display another automatic response to that threat. As a child this may be a tantrum or head banging. As an adult this could be getting drunk or self-harming, going on a spending spree, anything that will relieve the feeling brought about by the judgment of wrong or bad or stupid, even if it was our own judgment.

Meantime, we still have not found a correct response to the initial situation, and most likely have issued, along with others, yet another self-deprecating judgment about the second response, behaviour. And so it goes.

This is purely and simply because we did not judge the initial behaviour by the rules of simply effective or non-effective. This negative wheel occurred merely because we have developed low self-esteem and as a consequence we now habitually see ourselves in good/bad, right/wrong terms. We have been applying good/bad judgments, instead of accepting that is what is for reasons that were valid. Helpful or not that remains so. We did what we did for primarily valid reasons. There is no good/bad.

Earlier we talked about the labels that describe sets of commonly used behaviours. These labels are used to describe personalities and finally become the label attributed to the person them self. We used the examples of bossy, weak, clever. These labels attract a judgment measuring along the lines of good and bad. It is not just everybody else who applies these judgments through inference, it is us too. We do it, and we do it to ourselves.

The rate of judgment we apply to something is not always in the same place on the range of implication as it is to someone else. The range of good and bad is a measure after all. If you think of it in terms of a ruler, it may range from extremely bad one end, marked as 1 to extremely good the other end marked as 12. When someone attributes a personality describing word to us therefore, we attribute the actual measure we hold, not the measure they hold.

So, for example, if I held the belief that bossy is not very good at all, I may place it on my ruler as a 3. However, the person who had attributed the word bossy to me may not consider it to be so bad, so place it as a 5. Because I translate everything using my own ruler, (my own perspective), from that point on I will think the person that calls me bossy thinks of me as a 3 in terms of good and bad, even though they actually think of me as a 5.

These inferences of judgments add up. The point is if I have a particularly negative view of most things in life, my measures (my perspectives) are always going to be lower than someone who generally sees life in a more positive vein. Therefore I will then perceive others think much less of me than they actually do. This affects my self-esteem even more. I begin to suffer from even lower self-esteem. My own sense of self lowers as I build up a picture of how I believe I am perceived by the rest of the world, even though they don't actually view me that badly.

Low self-esteem affects our own judgmental scales with negative effect. We begin to get an even lower range of judging, and it becomes a downward spiral. It is true to say that most people suffering with low self-esteem feel others hold a view of them that is quite far removed from the truth in favor of the negative. Their measurements have been set by their own judgments, not those of the people around them.

A general lack of self-worth or value, a sense of hopelessness about and towards oneself in the context of life is most certainly classified as low self-esteem and causes depression. Negative self-criticism is destructive physically, emotionally and mentally, and as we have begun to realise it is also commonly unnecessary and untrue.

Bring yourself into the moment and see anew with an enquiring mind. Don't presume you know what others think, enquire with no expectation. See their responses as their responses, without your own negative glasses on. Think of the possibilities of translations of their response to you. Don't presume, don't pre-judge, don't think you already know, rather see anew. Actually come, see, as if for the very first time.

Social Acceptance

Self-perception and self-awareness are both necessary for successful integration into society. We are by nature social creatures. Continuing with our initial theme of survival, there is safety in numbers in terms of survival success. There is therefore a valid basic reason why we all want to be accepted and liked by others. It is in our make-up literally. We can pretend not to care what others think, but this is merely self-deception. We do care and we care for a good and valid reason.

Our acceptance into society and our acceptance of its rules has major implication both to ourselves and to others. Going back to our example of driving, we may have the ability to choose whether or not to keep within specified speed limits or which side of the road we drive on, and we may have the capability of altering our own actions according to that choice. However we also have the ability, to project our thoughts forward and think in terms of consequences.

To flout society's rules and regulations almost certainly results in undesirable consequences. These rules and regulations are given on the most part for our own benefit and for the benefit of those around us. They increase our chances of survival as a group, keeping us relatively safer on the roads or protecting us from haphazard predators.

When correcting our young for pulling another toddlers hair, we are establishing rules of behaviour that are beneficial to both our toddler and the other one. The girl with the long hair needs protecting from hurt and harm for no reason; our toddler's survival was not threatened by the girl with the long hair.

Our own child's self-esteem will not suffer as a result of this correction if the explanation and the surrounding information is given without judgment. If you show your toddler that the girl is nice and that he/she still gets the attention they require to feel safe, there will be no harm done by the correction. You will merely be pointing out what is. In this moment your child does have your love and attention, they are safe. The girl with the long hair is not as she was perceived by our toddler.

What harms self-esteem is when we are judged as individuals as wrong, or not nice, for no understandably valid reason in terms of effective or non-effective to survival. If judgment is needed at all, it becomes clear why we should be judging the action, not the individual; and why this judgment should most certainly be a measure of effective or not-effective, or even better a judgment of necessary against not necessary, not a judgment of good or bad. Communication should be that the unwanted behavioral response is not necessary or not effective in terms of survival. It needs to make sense in terms of what is.

Unhelpful judgments of children often arise through adult lack of information. Often parental responses are also instinctive reactions as opposed to informed choices.

If we don't initially judge our toddler as good or bad, but rather acknowledge the behaviour was an instinctive reaction that was most likely driven by his/her survival instincts, we can then begin to impart information, teach our youngster that in instances when they perceive fear, correctly or incorrectly, then another form of behaviour, will bring about a more beneficial response in terms of addressing and reducing the acknowledged feeling of fear. In real terms if you scold a child that is already fearful, you will add to its fear. By bringing about the disapproval of every large member of the social group that infants instinctive perceptions of its own chances of survival lessen, its fear increases. If we first identify the action as what it was, acknowledge that behaviour as appropriate in situations where survival is threatened, and then begin to add to our children's box of behavioral 'tools', as well as the vast array of ways to view life and its various circumstances, we enable them to begin to learn how to make informed and effective choices about and from the stable point of what is.

By utilizing our own appropriate and beneficial behaviours, by ourselves as parents making informed choices about our own responses to our children, we maintain our child's own self-esteem and increase their self-confidence.

As adults then, we have to learn to stop identify what this moment is actually about in terms of both our self and our circumstance, and then choose our own reactions, even with our own young. This also then maintains our own self esteem levels as well as increases our own efficiency in terms of raising a well-adjusted, happy child, who is confident in their own abilities. Our own offspring will then also have the knowledge and control to make individual informed choices without effort having accepted each moment from an unprejudiced viewpoint. That behaviour will also be automatic, because that is how their brain networks will develop.

This book isn't about how to raise your young. These principles are applicable to every social interaction we have. This is merely a prime example. Before we can teach our young to appreciate themselves, we have to learn to appreciate ourselves. We need to acknowledge our own needs within our own social communities, be they home, work or leisure. We need to identify our own actions and reactions (behaviours), acknowledge their purpose, throw away the bias and see each moment anew and then manage our self in terms of choosing which behaviour is going to be the most effective in that particular circumstance in bringing about the result we ultimately want to achieve.

There is no benefit to judging ourselves harshly. I cannot think of any situation in which debilitating self-judgment brings about a potentially desired result.

We are social creatures. Every piece of recovery literature in mental health acknowledges that human beings have a basic need to experience a sense of self-worth in, and acceptance from, the community, the social group in which they live.

This is instinctively linked to our own chances of survival. We don't acknowledge we are still reacting to those survival drives, but in actuality we all are. When we are able to acknowledge that, we stop beating ourselves up, stop feeling frustrated with ourselves, and cease endlessly asking the question 'Oh why did I do that!?'

We see, we acknowledge and then, only then, can we begin to manage our actions and reactions, our behaviours. Then we do become able to ensure we are effective at achieving the end results that we do want for each of our various life circumstances.

Realisation and Informed Choice

In summary so far, we have ascertained that from the deep recesses of our subconscious, we are all still being driven to behave in a certain way due to instinctive, deep seated drives based on the need to survive. Also we know we have learned rules and social behaviors. Sometimes we are able to modify instinctive behaviors, but many of our behaviours happen automatically in reaction to given cues. We don't consciously decide to do them.

At this point it is important to restate our basis. YOU do not need fixing. You were born perfectly equipped with instinct AND you have also learned other behaviours as well. You have both sets. In reality, you have more than two sets, you have many, but the point is, there is nothing to be fixed, nothing to be removed, you are not flawed. You have done as you were meant to do. You have multiple potential assets at your disposal, many behavioral tools in your tool box.

However, owning these tools does not necessarily bring quality of life. Merely having all these behaviours at the disposal of our subconscious can, as we have learned, bring discord and disharmony into our lives.

For example, if a dinner host is giving our partner the eye, flirting unreservedly, and we react with a behaviour typical of a stag in rut, we may realize from consequence that it was not the most effective way of keeping our spouse by our side throughout the dinner party, let alone for life. Whilst that behaviour may be highly effective in ensuring the continuum of our own genes when living in the forest, it is not likely to be effective in suburbia.

It is not enough to merely be capable of these behaviours. To utilize these assets effectively we need more. Three important ingredients we need to add are realisation, control and choice.

Firstly we need to realise our own automatic actions and reactions. We need to identify them.

Then we need to gain the ability to halt these automated responses long enough to make an informed choice. We need to be become aware in the moment. The result then becomes we perform a chosen response, rather than merely effect an automatic, non-chosen behaviour.

Due to the fact they have gone subconscious, we believe we have no control over many of our actions and reactions (behaviours). This is not the case.

Let's go back to our example of driving. Though having driven for many years it is an automatic behaviour, we do have the ability to control how we drive, where we drive, whether or not to indicate and even at what point we wish to change gear. We even have the control and the ability to choose which side of the road we drive on, how fast we will drive and whether or not we will keep to our society's rules of acceptable road behaviour.

If we have learned to drive on the right side of the road, it does take some thinking about when we need to drive on the left. We have developed many automatic responses when driving that ensure we keep to the rules of right side driving. These happen when we turn a corner, when we navigate a roundabout, when we choose a lane. Learning to drive on the left hand side of the road is about more than where we initially place our vehicle; it requires some active thought in each moment, as we drive.

However, as proved by the millions of people who hire cars on annual vacations to other countries, it can be done and relatively easily. Yes some effort and conscious thought has to be applied, but we are not talking immense difficulty here. It is relatively easy to accomplish and most definitely gets easier with practice! We know why. As we practice, our neurons grow more tendrils, that pathway becomes strengthened, and we don't have to consciously think about it all so much anymore.

The hardest part is the need to become aware of our automatic reaction to turn left at the roundabout, applying that initial conscious thought in that moment, thereby ensuring we choose the right lane and go right instead. It can be done.

We do have situations already where we prove to ourselves that altering an automatic behaviour can be done, and achieved in seconds. That process of 'aware, control, choose', happens in split seconds.

It is the same with our other behaviours. The minute we identify and apply control, we then have choice. We choose to turn left or right. We can choose how we act and react. We can identify and exercise control over our own responses and start making informed choices. We do not lose the original ability or choice to metaphorically drive on the left, we gain an ability to drive on the right also.

Again I will reiterate, we do not need fixing, we have not learned to drive incorrectly; we are learning something new and we are adding another choice. It is yet another tool in our toolbox.

We do not necessarily have to give up our present behaviors; it is highly likely most of them have been effective in prior circumstances. We merely need to empower ourselves to identify them in the cases where we wish we 'hadn't done that' at that particular time. We can then apply control and make a choice next time.

There are many benefits that come from being able to purposefully make these choices about our reactions, not least of which is the fact that the internal fight that causes us to feel so negatively about ourselves, the one that makes us feel so depressed or so useless, ceases to exist.

Once all sets of behaviours are accepted as what they are, effective or non-effective, for they all are in different situations and depending upon desired outcome, there is no internal conflict anymore. Conflict ceases to exist simply because you become the driver behind the behaviour, you make the choice. You cease being the victim.

This choice must be based on desired outcome and actual circumstance. It shouldn't be an instinctive survival response, nor should it be an 'I know I should do this, but I don't know why' response elicited by feelings or perceptions of judgment.

Each action and reaction must be seen without predetermined judgment. Each action and reaction must be known to bring its own benefits and its own disadvantages. There is no longer right and wrong, there is only the measurement of what is most helpful in the current circumstance. The decision is made in accordance with which behaviour is most likely to achieve the overall desired outcome we want. Instead of right or wrong, the measurement becomes about effective or non-effective and it is given in reaction to what actually is, not what we have pre-supposed.

Our human ability to gain knowledge and very quickly forecast consequences and results, gives us the ability to change simple choice into informed, therefore more potentially effective choice.

As mentioned earlier, meditation quietens our chaotic and predetermined mind. It develops mental culture. Mental culture aids awareness. Awareness reduces both danger and fear.

Control

When you first start these mind exercises, you do have to put in a bit of conscious thought. Once again it is good to realise that this is something you already possess; you do have the ability to think both consciously and sub-consciously. You can bring what is in the sub-conscious to the awareness of the conscious. You do this by becoming aware of how you are thinking, feeling and reacting in this moment. Conscious directed attention, that awareness of yourself in this moment, is what gives you the ability to apply control.

It really is simply a question of directing our conscious attention to the moment. When you do this, in neurological terms, you alter the neural pathways of your automatic responses so that they pass through your reasoning areas, your cognitive functions, namely your conscious awareness. You don't have to know how to do this, those neural networks will do it all by themselves. And no brain surgery is required. You just have to get in the habit of bringing your conscious attention to the now. The more you do it, the easier it becomes. It too will become automatic, habitual.

You gain control when you give yourself the chance to be aware of now. You give yourself the ability to think calmly and with clarity when you stop judging yourself; when you accept how you work and how you feel and acknowledge the valid reason for it. Without this judgment of good and bad, without that inner conflict, you are able to think in terms of effective or non-effective. If what you do is effective in bringing about your desired outcome, keep doing it. If it is not, stop and apply an alternative.

All this requires initially is time for reflection and time for meditation. I have suggested five minutes reflection a day as a discipline, just to get you 'in the habit'. Once your mind picks up on the habit, you will find yourself reflecting more often and for shorter periods. Remember we think extremely fast. You can have hundreds of thoughts in five minutes. Once you are in the habit of thinking this way, even if only for five minutes a day, you will begin to automatically become aware of and evaluate your own automatic responses at the time you do them. Your brain will begin to become aware in the moment it happens; because it will recognise and do preparation work in readiness for your prescribed five minutes. These processes happen in split seconds. You will start to automatically become aware in the precise moment you affect an automatic response, because you are literally training your brain to think in this way, to be aware of that element in that moment. You have changed the neural pathway, physically.

If you have ever attempted meditation, or practiced a relaxation programme, you may be aware that our thoughts have a tendency to run away with themselves often, follow their own path. Again this is habitual and caused by the formation of our neural pathways, one signal sending off multiple impulses. Those impulses will nearly always be picked up by the strongest neural networks. They have multiple tendrils; they are super sensitive to signal. Anything we have been constantly directing our attention to will be linked into many existing pathways, pinging our thoughts back to that subject at the slightest of prompts. Just remember that through non-use, these tendrils will die away. Our brains discard what we don't use. Again, no surgery is required. It is merely a case of controlling our thoughts, rather than letting our thoughts control us. This is aided by developing the art of Insight Meditation. When you begin the practice of meditation, again, begin slowly, five minutes if that suits and build it up. But make it a discipline. For five minutes, pay attention on purpose to this actual moment; how this moment really is in its entirety. What is your body doing? What is breathing like? How does your chair feel? What can you hear? Your mind will wander initially, simply acknowledge this and bring your attention back to your breathing, back to the feel of the chair, back to what you decide to place your attention on in this moment. That is mediation. Do it regularly and you will be astounded at the benefits.

We have often felt we have no choice about what we think. You may even think you are your thoughts. Let me prove to you this is not the case.

Get a piece of paper and a pen or pencil. Observe your thoughts for just a moment then write down what you were thinking, write down your thoughts. It doesn't matter what they are, you can throw the piece of paper away in a moment. No one will see it but you. Do that now.

Can you read what you have written? Now if you are your thoughts, how could you observe them? How could YOU know what your thoughts were thinking?

So you see you are not your thoughts. You are you. You have thoughts; you think. Most of your thoughts, most of the time are not in your conscious control, but they can be, when you want them to be. You wouldn't want them to be in your control all of the time. The object of this exercise is not to gain control of your thoughts all of the time. You only want to control your thoughts enough to gain control over your automatic responses when you want to. You only want to control your thoughts enough to question the beliefs that inhibit you. You only want to control your thoughts enough to change your perception when you choose to do so. You only want to control your thoughts enough to ensure the strong neural pathways in your brain are the ones you want them to be; the effective ones, the helpful ones, the happy ones. You want to remain master of your thoughts as opposed to constantly subjecting your existence to the effects of that habitual drudgery of preconceptions and prejudices.

Then you can leave your thoughts alone and have confidence in your own responses and enjoy your own multiple perceptions and experiences. Once your minds habits are the ones you want them to be, you have a new life, literally. The worries, the frustrations you presently have about you, go away.

Acknowledge Without Judgment

As mentioned, two major principles of Mindfulness Practice are 'Non-Judgment' and 'Acceptance'. We can link both these principles into the phrase 'acknowledge without judgment'.

Non judgment is a very difficult state to achieve and maintain. As discussed, we all judge all of the time. It is the judgment based on good/bad, right /wrong we are trying to avoid.

Acceptance may be perceived in many ways, e.g., acceptance of unacceptable behaviours, acceptance of anything that is given to us, acceptance of the situation we are in. Depending on the context, acceptance can seemingly portray many different things and it would be unwise, let alone impossible for us to say "yes, I accept I must be acceptant of all things".

So how do we in reality, acknowledge without judgment?

Let's consider two real life examples to explore this concept.

A couple of hours ago, I turned my heating system on. "It's so cold still", I said to my son in justification as I did so. That was a judgment. It was my judgment, and in continuing exploration of the power of language, it was actually spoken in an openly judgmental tone, propelled by my opinion that winter really should have been over some weeks ago. Fortunately for me, my son was also cold and so were most other people living in my home country of England. We had that year endured a hard winter that started early and finished late, that being a judgment measured against our cultural English method of seasonal timing, namely the month. By April, we expect it to be spring. The majority of us British were fed up with feeling cold, with scraping ice off our cars in the morning – in April! We all unashamedly spoke the same judgment. My judgment therefore was socially acceptable. The behaviour following that judgment, i.e. to turn the heating system on, was also received as socially acceptable. My son in the house with me likewise benefitted from the warmth the heating system brought, he was judging using the same range as I was. He was also feeling cold.

Now let's analyse this scenario under the lights of 'Acceptance' and 'Judgment', or more precisely 'acknowledge without judgment'.

I said "It's so cold". Firstly what is 'it'? What was I referring to, the environment, the weather, or me? Or indeed was I referring to any one of those things, all of them or none of them? In fact I was referring to none of them. I was referring to my own experience of my environment.

Hot and cold like so many areas of life are comparative, there is a range. I was having an experience I describe as feeling cold.

I was not physically cold. Had my body temperature been measured at the time, it would have been around 36.5C. My body was working perfectly and maintaining my optimal body temperature.

Inside my house at the time the temperature was around 12 degrees Celsius, quite warm compared to the temperature outside which was 3 degrees C, but which because of the wind chill factor, was confidently described by the national weather man as feeling like -1 degree C.

Due to all of these factors plus the poor state of my window and door fittings, my body was working hard to maintain my optimum body temperature. I 'felt' discomfort as my veins and arteries constricted in order to preserve heat. My neck and shoulder muscles were tensing evoking an overwhelming urge to cuddle myself, and the hairs on my skin were rising to provide me with an insulating layer of warm air. I felt driven to carry out an action that would assist in maintaining my optimum body temperature. The language centers within my brain acknowledged the communicative phrase that made this feeling recognizable to others in my social group. My behaviour, my set of reactions to the circumstance, was to say 'It's so cold' and turn on the heating. These behaviours all happened automatically within seconds, without me giving them any conscious thought.

So to acknowledge all this without judgment, I would when reflecting think, 'I acknowledge what my body was doing in response to environmental factors. I accept I communicated the feeling I experienced to my social group. I attempted to alleviate the discomfort I was feeling by initiating the heating system. It was successful, it was effective, and I did achieve my desired outcome of feeling warmer so I choose to affect that set of behaviors again.

If I wanted to change what happened, my only immediate choice is to change the two displayed behaviours. I cannot immediately change the temperature regulating mechanisms of my own physiology, but I may choose not to communicate my feeling to my social group. I may also choose to help myself feel warm or not. I may choose what to do to help myself feel warm. Another way for example would have been to put on more clothes. The circumstance is the circumstance. I cannot change the seasons, and in that instant, I could not change my window and door fittings.

So first we must accept the circumstance, the environment and then accept how that causes us to feel. We accept what is in that moment without judgment. Only from point of acceptance can we change it. If I try to change that circumstance from the point of for example 'Well it's April, it shouldn't be cold', I will move from a point I want to be at rather than from a point I am at. I may in that moment have remained cold, refusing to acknowledge what is as I habitually acknowledge instead, what I feel should be.

And I purposefully choose not to apply judgment when reflecting on this event. I acknowledge without judgment. I don't say, "Well I shouldn't be cold as it's not that cold". Nor did I say "I shouldn't have put the heating on as I cannot afford it". I simply acknowledged my environment, my feelings, my drives and my subsequent behaviors. I did not apply judgment in terms of right/wrong or good/bad.

Even if I could not afford the heating, I would say I initially put the heating on in response to feeling cold. However, as I have very little money, a more effective way of dealing with my problem may be to turn it off again and put more clothes on. I acknowledge that my primary instinctive behaviour in response to the cue 'feeling cold' was to turn on the heating, but I halt that default response momentarily, and choose to put more clothes on instead, consequently widening the range of effectiveness. Either way, I am not judging myself in terms of wrong and right, rather acknowledging what I did and acknowledging it was for valid reason, and then considering choice with a view of achieving the most effective outcome considering all my circumstances, i.e. in this case my financial circumstances as well.

I do employ techniques that help me to momentarily halt my automated reactions and give me the split seconds I need to make a choice. These are Mindfulness based reflection, relaxation and meditation exercises.

I still keep the choice to do as I did initially if I want to. I have lost nothing and I have fixed nothing. I have simply gained more abilities and they serve me well. I have increased my options, increased my choice.

So how do we acknowledge without judgment? The answer is simply by practice. As stated earlier, practice. Every day to start with take five minutes to reflect on what and who you have judged today in terms of right or wrong, good or bad. Acknowledge all facts to yourself openly and honestly. Do not attempt to justify to yourself, because without judgment there is no need. Weigh up options, alternative measures of judgments such as effective or non-effective, pleasurable or not so pleasurable, but at all costs practice avoiding the terms right, wrong, good or bad.

To start with you have to apply the conscious effort; you have to reflect on what happened for those five minutes. I guarantee that when something hasn't gone right, you will normally be spending more than five minutes a day thinking about it, so five minutes should not prove to be an impossible chore.

Also, these five minutes of planned reflection won't need to happen for long. After a few days of doing this planned practice, you will notice yourself becoming aware in the moment of such times where you have applied right/wrong or good/bad judgment. Your mind will automatically begin to do this for you in preparation of your planned five minute reflections, purely because you are doing it regularly. You will also notice you have automatically increased your own toolbox of measuring tools. Rather than right/wrong, you will begin to measure in many alternative ways, effective or not effective particularly and therefore not judging yourself or others so harshly.

We think exceedingly fast and soon, as this practice becomes habitual, as it too goes automatic, you will not need to consciously spend five minutes performing this exercise. You will notice that you are recognizing when you judge in the moment you judge and counteracting it automatically on each occasion it happens.

Take great pleasure in this achievement because you have effectively carried out Cognitive Behavioural Therapy (CBT) on yourself. You have physically altered your neural pathways. Were you able to do brain scans on yourself before and after, you could literally see this change in neural networking.

This is a magnificent achievement. Make sure you recognise and acknowledge that. You are now well on the path to being able to automatically choose how you want to behave in the moment. You are now beginning to control your own thinking habits and therefore your own reactions.

In actuality we do all reflect every day. It is just that making this a positive decision, making this a planned event rather than a haphazard one where your habitual thoughts take the reins, helps your mental culture. It assists you to work with the natural inclinations of your own mind without becoming victim to them.

Keep up with the meditation though. Even if you only manage five minutes a day, take five minutes to close your eyes and train your mind to pay attention on this moment, to see anew, to experience for the first time everything you think you have experienced a million times before. I don't expect you will stay at five minutes. Quality meditation brings about such a relaxed state that you will want to be there for more than five minutes.

Regular meditation is proven to have spectacularly positive results. Research shows its benefits to heart and circulatory systems, the immune system, quality of sleep, improved concentration, improved cognitive functioning.

Mindful Meditation teaches you how to disentangle yourself from your habitual cognitive thought processes. It is the mental art of stepping out of your own way. The discipline of mediation is the key to mental and emotional culture. Through the regular practise of Mindful Meditation we give ourselves the chance to behave in an ethical and helpful manner in daily life. Ethical and helpful behaviour does not follow hard and fast rules because it is dictated by authority, rather it becomes chosen and enacted because it is the most beneficial according to the needs of each situation that arises in our day to day existence.

Making helpful choices regarding our behaviours, requires an ability to be aware of all or as many of the factors in every situation as possible and to then carry out a unique, creative and appropriate response each time. It is the ability to choose a precise set of actions which will be truly optimal in each daily situation. If you try to juggle all the information involved in this every time a situation arises using your cognitive conscious mind, you'd wear yourself out. Luckily a deeper level of our consciousness does this processing with ease. Through regular meditation, we give the vast libraries of our subconscious a chance to flow. We quiet the incessant nattering thoughts of our habitual conscious, and give ourselves equal access to all parts of our mind brain. Regular meditation equals regular flow time. It is that simple. The more you meditate, the more you access all of your mind's current potential.

Challenging Your Perceptions and Beliefs

A great way of realizing what colors your own perception of life is by utilizing Cognitive Behavioural Therapy (CBT). Of course there is much more to CBT. The aim of this book is to convey some of the principles of various approaches, therapies and practices. Were I to go into each one in detail, this book would be huge.

However, much benefit can be gained from developing your knowledge about all these different ways of helping yourself. Supplying your brain with more information gives it, therefore you, more options to choose from. Remember this is about increasing your choices.

Working with a Cognitive Behavioural Therapist on a one to one basis is extremely helpful in identifying schemas and filters that actually affect how you perceive yourself and the world around you. If you have the resources to do this, do it. You will be amazed at the thousands of beliefs dictating your perceptions and therefore your behaviours.

Alternatively there is self-help literature or talking books and either CD or web based programs if you are not an avid reader.

Meantime, this book will give you an overview and an understanding of what is meant by schemas and filters.

All human beings live a subjective experience, not a factual one. All of our own experiences are exactly that, our own experience. We can in actuality all 'experience' the same circumstance, however our own perception of it guarantees it will be a completely unique experience.

We have seen that our perceptions are greatly influenced by our own judgments, and our own reactions, and vice versa. However they are also highly influenced by our own beliefs.

As we have learned, most judgmental measuring tools are comparative. Where various things are placed within the range on our own personal measuring tools, depends largely upon our own experience and our own perceptions. We have already used the example of hot and cold and bossy. We could also apply the same principles to fast and slow, and almost everything else!

Our own experience largely dictates our own beliefs. Using the fast/slow example, this is how beliefs also affect our judgments, our perceptions and therefore our subsequent behaviours.

Hundreds of years ago, before the onset of machinery, the fastest thing humans in England may have known about or experienced in one way or another, would have been a horse. It would have been fair enough for them to describe their experience of riding a running horse as going extremely fast. The end range of their measure would be the limit of what they know, plus a bit. To travel over 200 miles an hour would have been inconceivable a couple of hundred years ago. Even more so, if you were to try to convey that concept to a caveman, he would simply think you are mad, because his belief about what is possible and what is not would simply have dictated that it is impossible. His belief system would not accept that as fact.

To a large extent we believe what we see. This is extremely limiting. The BBC documentary 'Invisible World', narrated by Richard Hammond, shows just how limited our vision is. The blink of an eye takes 50 milliseconds; it takes the brain 150 milliseconds to process what we see. This creates a time lapse, however tiny. Everything that happens during this time lapse and many things do, we simply do not see. If you were told about the myriads of things happening around us at any given time, without having seen this documentary, made possible using high speed filming technology, you simply would not believe them.

Our total knowledge of possibilities plus a little dictates to a large extent our beliefs. If someone came and told you they had been time travelling, and just come back from Egypt in the year 600BC, you would accuse them of being mad or lying, because your total knowledge plus a bit decrees your belief that this is not possible. In order for you to believe them, they would have to provide you with more knowledge, which always comes from an experience of sorts, even if it is reading or hearing it. Even on reading or hearing it, if the new knowledge conflicted with your current perception of factual knowledge, (your beliefs), you would still not readily accept it. A belief is something that is accepted as a fact.

Even our own lived experiences need to be backed up by our own belief system if we are to accept them.

Have you ever had a 'strange' experience? We may call these experiences spiritual, psychic or other-worldly, but we question whether we actually had that experience at all. Often the furthest we will go in acceptance of that experience is to tell ourselves we must have imagined or dreamt it. Unless it falls in with our own belief system we do not readily accept even our own lived experience.

Beliefs are extremely powerful and they not only color our perceptions, they dictate largely how we live. They have massive influence on our potential experience because we simply live within our own belief system.

When we speak of beliefs we tend to jump to thoughts of religion. Beliefs are about everyday life, you physically live by them. They are anything you consider to be fact.

You have infinite belief in gravity pulling you to the ground. You automatically account for its effects when you move. You limit your actions in line with this belief in gravity. You do not ever try to jump to the top of a ten storey building, purely because you accept as fact, believe, you cannot.

You believe you have a limited potential. Most of us don't try for magnificent wealth beyond taking a chance with the lottery, because we believe we will not be able. We do not apply for jobs we may like to do because we believe we will not be successful. We simply, on the most part, do not try to do anything that is against our own belief of possibility.

If you have ever seen the film the Matrix, this brilliantly conveys just how powerful our belief system really is, and it is true. Neo did not believe he was part of a computer system, so he could not jump off the top of one building and seemingly fly to another. In order to become successful, in order to be able to keep up with Trinity, he had to alter his belief; he had to accept, believe, to know without doubt that he was part of a computer programme, even though it felt like his experience of the real world as he knew it.

We do not attempt many things we could in reality achieve because we believe we will not succeed, or we believe we cannot. I have many times nursed individuals who have become hospitalized as their anxiety has caused them to believe they cannot carry out daily functions. And all the time they truly believe they can't, they can't. They do stop themselves.

We also have very strong beliefs about our own perceptions; we believe things are as we see them, when actually on closer examination, they are not. We may believe we are not beautiful, when actually we are to someone. Many of us believe we are bad or useless, when actually we definitely are not, as hopefully you have seen.

The point being, we are living our daily lives in accordance with these beliefs, limiting our own potential, and thereby actually creating our own reality, our own existence.

We do not believe we are in control of our own actions half the time, when now hopefully, I am altering your belief through knowledge and showing you that you are or at least that you can be.

We each hold hundreds of thousands of individual beliefs that color and filter our perceptions and subsequently control so many of our actions.

There have been amazing TV documentaries showing that we do not even see things that are there if we do not believe they can be there. If they do not fall in with our own belief about the norm, about the accepted, we simply do not even register them. We even 'filter' our own sensory experiences! Our brains do not process everything our senses take in. Many signals are discarded as irrelevant because they do not fall in with our own beliefs about what actually is, and also about what is relevant. These beliefs are so deep within us we are not even aware we hold them.

Time with an effective Cognitive Behavioural Therapist would surface amazing facts about your own personal beliefs and most certainly empower you to manage your own life more in keeping with your own wishes.

The practice of Mindfulness enables you to see what is, escape the limitations of your own prejudices and current beliefs.

Beliefs dictate outcomes and therefore society also bombards us with potentially false beliefs. Advertisers and politicians are masters of it. So is the media. Most of us know we should not believe what we read in the papers, but most of us still do. If the media tells us there will be a fuel shortage, most of us believe them enough to rush out and queue for two hours at the nearest fuel station to ensure we get some of what we now believe is left. Our actions as a result of our beliefs create a fuel shortage, however temporary. When it turns out to be nothing more than a political or economic hoax, most of us go round believing we must be stupid because we don't know what or who to believe anymore. However our belief in our political system and our own media system is still so strong that we will do it again next time, even if we have to pacify ourselves with the phrase 'just in case'. Beliefs have an astounding impact on our lives.

Every single self-motivational book or presentation will target your belief system. There are some brilliant ones about and I recommend you spend time seeing just what is out there. Beliefs have either an amazingly inspirational or a devastatingly limiting effect on us and consequently on our life.

Any good salesman knows he has to believe he will make the sale in order to be successful. Winston Churchill's speech given to the troops just before they embarked on their mission to Dunkirk was highly motivational in that he instilled in them (and very effectively) the belief that they would win, they would succeed. They believed him and they did despite factual odds in terms of numbers and weather being against them. He rationalized success in terms of commonly held and deep seated beliefs. They genuinely believed there was no alternative; they went out knowing they would win. This in turn highly influenced their actions.

When you have mastered the art of acknowledging without judgment, practice the same exercise on your belief system. Spend five minutes every day challenging, questioning everything you believe, namely everything you accept as fact. Now when I say everything, I mean everything you accept as a fact. Remember neural pathways increase with use, decrease through non-use. Make questioning what you accept as fact an automatic behaviour. Apply a few days of conscious thought, use the five minutes a day system, the rest will happen automatically, your body and mind are amazing.

When you challenge or question your beliefs, do it without intention and without expectation. Do not intend to find things you don't believe in. As you question what you accept as fact, many things on closer examination you will still accept as factual. That's ok; you are not doing it wrong. However what you will notice is that some things are not quite as definite on appraisal as you first thought. Many things will be recognised as comparative rather than factual.

We have already explored this concept when we discussed me saying 'It's so cold'. Did I hold the belief it was cold? Yes I did. And was it cold? Yes it was. However it was not an actual fact that I was cold. My temperature was normal body temperature but I was feeling the discomfort my body was experiencing to keep it at normal temperature. And even though the same factual elements were there for my son, he may not have felt as cold as I did. You will begin to notice that many of our beliefs are about things that actually are comparative; they have little to do with hard and fast facts.

As you do this exercise, pay close attention to beliefs you have about yourself. You may think it is a fact that you are overweight for example, or too thin. I am not expecting you to talk yourself out of this belief. I am asking you to explore whether you really deep down believe it. Too fat or thin for what? Too fat or thin compared against what? Too fat or thin in whose opinion?

As you think about this you may realise that actually your own belief is that you are too fat or too thin in a lot of other people's opinion. However surprisingly you may not totally hold the same belief. For example, I may on examination find that I acknowledge I am overweight when looking at the national BMI (body mass index) scale, but I do not actually believe I am TOO fat for what I want to do or accomplish or be. On reflection, I may realise I do not believe I am not too fat for my own desired end result. If that is the case, that may explain why I am unsuccessful when I diet. I have a deep seated belief that I am not **too** fat even though I acknowledge some other people may think I am. My own belief will definitively affect my actions and therefore my chances of success if and when I attempt to diet. I will be dieting against my own belief system and unless I change that belief, I am not likely to be any more successful than Neo was when he first tried to jump off the building.

My intention is not to influence your appraisals of your own beliefs in any way. The important thing is that you are honest with yourself and honest without judgment. Realise in this exercise that you do not have to believe what other's believe. This exercise is about you realizing just what you really believe, how you really think.

Are what you accept as facts, really facts?

At times this exercise is extremely liberating. Having spent the last few years skulking round trying to be invisible because you feel others perceive you as too fat, and finding that actually you do not believe you are too fat, you get a surge of confidence, a sense of release and liberation. In whatever area you find this experience, enjoy that feeling. It is yours, experience it with self-pride and savour it. Live that moment. Realise how much wider your own scope of experience has now become. Realise how many more choices have just opened up to you, simply because you challenged a belief.

Is there something in life you would really like to do? Why you don't do it? Do you hold the belief that you can't? Do you hold the belief that you will never be able? Do you currently not even try? Do you currently dismiss this desire? If so, question it. Is it really true? Is it a totally unquestionable fact that you will never be able? Are there factually no possibilities whatsoever? I am not asking if it is likely or unlikely, I am asking is it factually true that you could never achieve this desired result? If on reflection you find this is not fact, it was just your current belief; the result is your mind will now be open to accepting possibilities in line with this desire. Your mind will now be open to physically 'see' things already around you that could assist in facilitating this dream, this desire. Remember, you do not see that which does not fall in line with your own belief system. If there is a doubt about your belief, don't you owe it to yourself to open up the world of potential, the world of possibility that is already there? If you do this you lose nothing. If you do this, you just open up the possibility for more choices, more options and more rewarding experiences.

Then take this a step further. If you think your own real belief is not the same as the majority of others, question that belief. Ask why? If you believe others think differently – question that. Ask - do they really? Why do you believe that? Is it actually factual? Why are there differences in what we believe? If it is fact for me, why is it not fact for him/her? Is there a possibility this is not a belief but an opinion? What upholds my opinion? What proof is there of my beliefs?

When we hold a belief about ourselves that we do believe to be factual, we presume others hold the same belief about us.

We discussed earlier that our experiences are totally unique. That applies to every experience we have. The mechanics and subsequent actions of all of our sensory systems are unique. When we 'see' something, all the varying mechanics of our optical system whilst generally working on the same principles as everyone else's are totally unique. The chemical and electrical 'messages' our brain receives when we 'see' have to be interpreted. Our brains all interpret differently. There is no way so far to prove that when you see the colour yellow, you are having the same experience of yellow that I am.

This applies to everything in life. Life is a unique experience lived by our own perception of absolutely everything, yet we presume others have the same experience. The truth is that sometimes others experience similarly but never ever do they experience the same. That is something worth remembering next time you want someone to agree with you. We constantly seek reassurance and confirmation of our experiences, but actually in total we can never factually obtain them. It is impossible. The whole of life, everything you see, feel, hear, taste, touch, smell is your perception, my perception, their perception. It is never ever totally, wholly the same.

It stands to reason therefore, that to take this to the furthest extent, beliefs can never be total. They will always be to the individual best of our knowledge and experience thus far. The cave-man did not believe we could travel through the air at six hundred miles an hour, and at the same time have the experience of being still. Thousands of years later we are able to believe this because our increased knowledge and our own experience, even if we have not personally been on an airplane, allow us to believe it.

Our beliefs are limited by our own experience and no-one ever has the same experience. That is a thought worth contemplating. That is a thought well worth bringing to mind next time you are upset or unhappy or stressed or uncomfortable. Question your beliefs about that situation. Are they limited? Wonder about the next person's belief about that same situation. Lose the expectation that they will totally know how you perceive this experience, and lose the belief that you know how they feel. You don't, you can only imagine it in keeping with your own experiences, your own perceptions. The same applies to them for you.

Life is totally a perception. When you use a different comparative measuring scale, it appears you are changing the facts. What you are doing is changing your perception of the facts, and that in turn changes your experience. If you choose to use a different measuring scale, or a different filter, you are choosing to and accomplishing changing your experience of life. External factors do not change, however your experience of those external factors may change dramatically.

If you do the exercises suggested, your experiences will change noticeably. You will open yourself up to a world of possibility literally. You will begin to see things that have always been there, but you never noticed before. You will begin to be able to experience multiple perceptions of the same circumstance. Again, this is about choice. Stay where you are if you want to. You do not have to move, it is your choice. Keep your current perception if you want to, that is your choice. However, I recommend you at least try some others, at least then you know you really do have a choice. You don't lose the ones you had.

So how do you choose an alternative perception within the same circumstances?

I once read a brilliant example in a book called 'The Enlightened Response' by Ross Page. Lets' set the scene, the external circumstances you can do nothing about.

Your alarm did not go off. You are going to be late for work. You have to drive five miles to work and there are road works going on. The fact remains you are going to be late for work and this is going to be noticed by your boss.

Experience 1. You jump out of bed in a state of panic. In your haste you jump into the shower before the cold water has a chance to mix with the hot water and scold yourself. By the time you are dressed, your heart is pumping, you are not thinking clearly, hence you cannot remember where you left your keys. You are in panic and you feel horrible. You physically have evoked your own fight/flight response, even though your survival is not threatened. What a way to start the day. You finally find your keys, get in your car, zoom off down the road, and begin to wonder if you turned off the plugs. You know full well round the corner, the road works commence and you are going nowhere fast for the next two miles. An internal fight has begun in you. Should you go back to check the plugs or should you just keep going? You are on the edge of your seat, wishing the car in front of you would go just a little faster before the lights change to red again, but no; he doesn't. You are tapping the steering wheel, feeling really agitated now. The whole thing is a nightmare. You finally arrive at work, an hour late and feeling nauseous, stressed and worried. You catch one glance of your boss's stern face, and all the anxiety rushes out in a torrent of defensive words and most likely some underlying abuse. You feel like you hate the man. It wasn't your fault the alarm did not go off, why does he have to be so punitive? The atmosphere between the two of you remains tense all day. You make multiple errors because the stress and tension has affected your concentration and performance. You hate yourself for making things worse, convincing yourself by the end of the day that you will probably get sacked soon anyway. Your mind ruminates on it all. By lunchtime you have a thumping headache, need to go to the chemist and forget to buy a new alarm clock. The day just goes from bad to worse.

Ring any bells?

Experience 2. The exact same external circumstances apply. Your alarm does not go off, so you wake up later than you should. You acknowledge you are going to be late for work; you acknowledge you cannot turn back the time. You accept the best choice is to get showered and dressed as quickly as you can but without making matters worse, (hence you do not scold yourself). You carry out your normal routine of checking that all the plugs are turned off. In your calm state of mind you remember exactly where you put your keys last night and you begin your drive to work knowing full well there are road works just around the corner. You think to yourself, as I am going nowhere fast for the next two miles, I may as well listen to that new CD I bought yesterday. As you do this, you notice the sun is shining which makes you smile. You open the sunroof and relax back in your seat, knowing that for the next two miles, however long it takes, you are sitting in the sun listening to your new CD. You arrive at work knowing you are late and accepting your boss has to note this. You notice his frown as you walk in, but acknowledge him respectfully, apologize for being late, accept he has to say something about it, and make a mental note to buy a new alarm clock in your lunch hour so it doesn't happen again. Meanwhile you reflect on how enjoyable it was sitting in the sun this morning, you didn't expect to be able to do that today. That has put you in a good relaxed frame of mind and you get on with your day performing your job well and chatting to the boss as normal.

So nothing changed externally. However in Experience 2, you accepted, and acknowledged the facts without judgment. You acknowledged it was not your fault and you allowed yourself to make the most of the situation that was. Through the road works, instead of your thoughts racing ahead to a confrontation, you remained in the moment and enjoyed what that moment could bring, namely sunshine and good music. Even though you are late for work, you acknowledge you are working effectively to address that and there was good to be had here and now, in the meantime, in this moment. You accepted the job your boss had to do, knowing if you were in his position, you would have to do it also. You therefore made it as easy for him as you could, which in turn reduced the negative impact that had on both you and him. You remained calm, performed well and enjoyed your bosses company as normal for the rest of the day. You were able to purchase a new alarm clock in your lunch hour, thereby reducing the chance of that external circumstance happening again.

We do have the choice how to live each moment. Sometimes there is nothing we can do to alter external circumstances. Sometimes external circumstances are not helpful. However, there is nearly always good to be found in each moment if you choose to see and choose to allow it.

How you perceive things will affect your biological responses, and they will affect your ongoing circumstances. If you accept your boss as a man with a job to do, he is more likely to understand the alarm didn't go off. If you choose to perceive him as an enemy, a threat, a predator, it is highly likely you will evoke your own fight/flight responses, and also his. As you cannot fight or run in that situation, you are both highly likely to end up stressed.

How you experience each situation can be about choice. Bringing your attention to the moment, seeing all there is to see, then choosing your perception changes your lived experience. It really is that simple.

The Wisdom of Emotion

So here we are, at this point, accepting we are where we are. How do we know which way to go, how do we know which response to choose?

Largely we will use our knowledge, project our thoughts forward into consequences and choose the option most likely to bring about the most desirable outcome. But when we don't know, when we do not yet have that knowledge or the facts seem confusing or unsolvable; or deep inside, we know what we should do, but we just can't; which way do we go? How do we know?

It's easy. As Esther Hicks went on to say, we have our own internal guidance system. We have our own inbuilt ready-made navigation system. It's called feeling. It signals through emotion.

Have you ever said I wish I didn't feel this way? Have you ever said I feel down? Have you ever said I don't feel good today? Have you ever felt I should, but I simply don't want to?

Alternatively, have you ever thought I feel really good about this? Have you ever felt like you were on the top of the world? Have you ever felt excited or inspired? Or, this makes no sense, but I feel grand?

Well that is it. Start listening. Either way, feeling up or feeling down, have confidence in how you are feeling, because guess what? – It is right.

Has that shocked you? See even your own feelings don't need fixing. They are doing a grand job; they are desperately trying to tell you something is wrong if they are negative, or that something is just the way it should be if they are positive.

If you feel badly about something, your feelings are trying to warn you that some mismatch is occurring. What you should do is listen to them, heed the warning, acknowledge and accept it really is there for a good and valid reason.

You are not broken, you are working perfectly; you are just not listening. You are trying to ignore your very own perfectly working guidance system. It is now you need to look to your thoughts and follow your feelings. What is worrying you? What is your mind ruminating on? What keeps bubbling to the surface? What is causing this dissent, this internal struggle?

Listen without judgment. As you did earlier, listen to your thoughts awhile; write them down if it helps. Where are they going? Do they keep returning to a certain thing? If so, these are the things that require your conscious attention. They do not require your judgment, they require your understanding and your compassion.

Do you keep feeling bad when you think you shouldn't? Then listen because these are the areas where you need to consciously assess your judgments, your perceptions and your beliefs; your own body, mind and emotions are trying to tell you that.

Just as you have done before in the previous exercises, ask yourself: - What do I believe about this thing my mind is fixed on? Is what I believe actually true? Am I limiting myself? Can I change the way I perceive this thing? Can I experience it in a different way? Do I perceive this worry the same way as others or am I just presuming I do? If I take their chair, if I stand in their shoes, would I feel as I am feeling now? Has ruminating simply become a habit of mine that is no longer effective?

Did you react today in a way you didn't want to? If yes, this is what you need to consciously think about now in this same way. Did you get upset today? If yes, this is what you need to bring into conscious control now. Reflect, observe and acknowledge how you felt. Maybe you don't know exactly why you felt that way, but acknowledge that you did. Know that you felt this way for a perfectly valid reason, even if you don't know what that reason is just now. To continue feeling that way is not helpful, so change it. What is the next best feeling? What one single thought can you have right in this moment to feel slightly better? What in this moment along with all the turmoil, haven't you noticed yet?

Don't expect to go from totally miserable to ecstatically happy in 60 seconds, just take the first step. Allow yourself to go from feeling totally miserable to slightly sad. Go from slightly sad to ok. Go from ok to content. What one step makes you feel slightly better? Put your conscious thought into achieving that one step and do it honestly. Be true to yourself. If at this moment you feel that crying your eyes out will make you feel a bit better, do it. Allow yourself that, acknowledge without judgment. Your body and mind know themselves, stop fighting, stop resisting; begin allowing and follow the signs to the next step, the next slightly better feeling. That next best feeling is your map to happiness, follow it one step at a time, listening to yourself all the way, acknowledging without judgment each moment along the way.

If you absolutely hate someone in this very moment, don't expect yourself to love them within 60 seconds. Take the first step only. Will changing hate to dislike make you feel better? Will changing hate to contempt feel slightly better. If so do it. Change your perception of that circumstance just enough. Allow yourself to feel slightly better. Allow yourself to accept just one saving grace about that person just for a moment IF the feeling is slightly better. Or feel anger if that feels better. Trust your feelings in this instance. Allow them to guide you to a better state of mind, a better way of feeling. This is your very own guidance system. It works, it doesn't need fixing; you just have to allow it to work. Don't escape the feeling; don't blur it under a flood of alcohol or sedatives, as it will still be there later. Acknowledge it without judgment and allow it to evolve into its next state. Don't hinder that process.

This is all you ever have to do. You only ever have to take that first step. When you have done that you have succeeded. If you want to take it further this afternoon or tomorrow or next month, then fine, think about that this afternoon, tomorrow or next month. And when and if you do, that is the first step again. All you have to do at the time you choose is consciously choose that first step. The rest will happen.

Sometimes when we reflect on something that has been upsetting, our minds may tend to ruminate. People suffering from depression often suffer this symptom; their thoughts get stuck on an unpleasant issue that seems to replay over and over in the mind like a broken record, or a computer with an unsolvable puzzle. This may feel like your head just won't let go.

If this happens, acknowledge the issue that is worrying you, but also acknowledge there is no answer at this point, if this is the case. Then consciously move your thoughts to something else. It is likely your mind will find its way back. That's ok, don't fight yourself. Acknowledge the situation is literally playing on your mind, again accept there is nothing you can do in this moment if that is the case and gently move your thoughts onto something else again, something that makes you feel better, even if only slightly better. This is conscious control, but it is important it is not forced, just firm and gentle. Allow, acknowledge and then move. If it is persistent, if the ruminating continues, use distraction techniques that work for you. A general guide for positive distraction is something you enjoy that takes your attention. However, remember the neural pathway in use is going to be strengthened with use. Acknowledge to yourself that ruminating is not helping. Acknowledge it does not feel good. Accept what your mind is doing, accept it is doing it for valid reason, but gently, firmly move your thoughts on. It will get easier. These types of worry tend to evaporate after a while, or alternatively when the mind is at peace, an answer presents itself. Just bring yourself into this moment, because this moment is all you need to deal with right now. Know you will take action when you can, when circumstances allow. This is not a case of accepting this forevermore, it is a case of accepting that this is where you are right now, and these are the available choices right now. It is about allowing the good into this moment, not just the bad.

The same applies to positive feelings, positive emotions. If you are feeling happy, good, loved, any positive emotion, take note of it. Revel in it. Think about what is causing this feeling and make sure you consciously do it again. So often we only notice the negative times. Are you feeling excited about something? That is great. You are literally physically prepared for a wonderful experience; your system is expecting it. Have you ever felt inspired? Do it, go with that flow. Make the most of this moment.

Also, take the time to notice how you feel when you are simply ok. Notice you actually feel ok most of the time. Notice how Ok feels. Actually Ok in this life of worry and frustration can feel good. Notice the sunshine. If you live where I live, we don't see it often, and when we do it simply makes us feel so good; everyone literally starts smiling. Notice the wonder of nature going on around you. Notice the clouds in the sky. Notice the birds singing. Think about someone you love. Think about someone who makes you laugh. Notice all that feels so nice in your life. Notice that as you direct your attention, your thoughts, on purpose, the affect it has on how you feel in this moment. Come, see again this moment. Experience it now with that new feeling, that new perspective, that new thought. Consciously experience each experience again and again and you will understand about seeing anew. Don't let the nice things in life slip by unnoticed. Help them become habitual.

Positive emotions feel good. They are also physically good for you. They have the opposite effect to stress. We all notice both the physical skip in our step, the increase in energy levels and the esoteric high we experience when we feel love. This is the opposite of stress in all ways. This is physically good for us.

Gratitude and appreciation are also positive emotions and when we are truly grateful for something we literally feel that warm glow. Feeling and showing gratitude and appreciation is something that is very much in our own control. All too often we take things for granted and forget to notice and to be thankful. I guarantee if you make an effort to display gratitude and appreciation for as many things as you can, each and every day, you will be amazed at how good you feel, at how much your mood lifts and how much your energy levels increase. It is so simple yet so effective.

You are in ultimate control of your thoughts, as and when you choose to be. Your thoughts have direct effect on your feelings. Your feelings also have direct effect on your thoughts. Your thoughts and feelings ultimately affect your physical wellbeing also. It is a circle. Which way the circle turns is up to you.

Do not become victim to your thoughts, as you have learned not to become the victim of your automatic responses. Purposefully direct your thoughts toward the positive things in your life. They are there; you just have to notice them. Do not become victim to persistent negative feelings. Acknowledge them, know why they are there and choose to change them. You can be happy if you simply choose to be.

All the little things count, they all add up to either a negative or positive slant on your existence, your life. This is in your control. Your mind and body work for you. If you look after them, they will look after you.

Food For Thought ... and Water

It is simply impossible to write a book about looking after your mind and body without referring to dietary intake. It does have an impact. We have seen how emotion, physiology and thought are all inextricably linked. Therefore what you eat, the things you introduce into your physical system will affect how you feel physically, therefore how you feel emotionally, and in turn will affect your thoughts.

I am not going to tell you don't eat this, don't eat that. That information abounds all around us, but it doesn't necessarily motivate us into choosing wisely.

However, I would be letting you down if didn't say what is going to impact on your mental wellbeing. Put simply it would be the same as me telling you how to get the best out of your car, without letting you know what fuel you should put in it.

Research shows that there are fewer cases of anxiety and depression in the Southern Mediterranean countries than Northern Europe. This research suggests this could be due to higher intakes of fish and olive oil and less red meat and dairy products. There is also lower consumption of processed foods and more fresh fruit and vegetables. The authors of a Spanish study into this propose it is due to a synergistic combination of omega 3 fatty acids together with other natural unsaturated fatty acids and antioxidants from olive oil and nuts. It is thought that flavonoids and other phytochemicals from fruit and other plant foods together with large amounts of natural folates and other B vitamins in the common Mediterranean diet provide a fair degree of protection against depression. Omega 3 fish oil is now often prescribed in mental health practice. Put simply, fish, nuts, fresh fruit and vegetables and less of the microwave ready can positively affect your mental and physical wellbeing. Remember it is the circle, physical, emotional, mental. Whatever you do to improve one will have a positive knock on effect to the others.

Studies link depression with low levels of the mineral selenium. The recommended daily amount is 0.075mg for men and 0.06mg for women. Brazil nuts are a good source of selenium, providing one third of women's RDA in each nut. Unrefined grains, cereals, meat, and eggs are also good sources of selenium. So now we are adding some meat, eggs, grains and cereals and keeping with the nuts.

Choosing slow release carbohydrates and foods that are slow to digest for energy rather than sugary foods, prevents sugar rushes that are commonly followed by energy slumps. Blood sugar levels are known to affect mood, with moods shown to fluctuate up and down with the blood sugar levels. Choose foods with a low GI (glycaemic index) such as oats and bran cereals, beans, pulses and lentils as well as apples and oranges. In summary, we are going with the foods we listed above.

Protein and tryptophan-rich foods – such as chicken and turkey, tuna and salmon, beans and seeds can be most effective when eaten alongside slow-release carbohydrates. This is because tryptophan is converted by our bodies into serotonin. Lack of available serotonin in neural synapses is thought to be the major cause of depression. Most anti-depressant medications target serotonin levels. The blood-to-brain absorption of tryptophan is helped by carbohydrates. It makes simple sense. In terms of everyday food, now we have added some poultry.

Turmeric added to foods is said to supply directly to the mitochondria in cells. Mitochondria are the energy factories of cells, so this would enhance energy at cellular level.

There is plenty of information around the five-a-day principle as well as avoiding high cholesterol and high salt content foods that eventually inhibit circulation and are a major cause of heart disease.

The above lists a range of commonly eaten foods. It isn't difficult; to me it shouts balance of basic food types. Living on burgers, chocolate, oven chips and take-away isn't going to do you any physical (or mental, or emotional) favours.

And drink! Put simply no other nutrient is more essential or is needed in such large amounts as water. It is needed in our cells, around our cells. It is needed to transport nutrients around our bodies. We use it as cushioning internally. Our bodies are around 60% water, our brain and muscle being 75% water. I don't know how many times I have heard people say 'oh but I don't like water'. What's to like or not like? It's a bit like saying I don't like air (in my opinion). This one time I feel inspired to say - Just do it. Trust me on this one, simply having a glass of plain water a day or throughout the day, supplementing the fluids that you do like, will make you feel a whole lot better.

Put simply the performance of our bodies and minds are affected by what we do or don't put into them.

Exercise

We all know that exercise is important, but do we know why? What sort of exercise, how much? Nearly all of us walk around during the day or wander up the shop once a week; is this enough? Not all of us want to look like a body-builder, so how much exercise is enough?

Basically there are two types of exercise, aerobic and anaerobic. Aerobic simply means 'with oxygen'; anaerobic means 'without oxygen'. The two types of exercise differ by the intensity of muscle activity and also by how the muscle produces energy.

Aerobic exercise is necessary for a number of reasons. It strengthens the respiratory muscles, the ones you use to breathe. It strengthens the heart muscle, maintaining or improving its ability to pump blood around your body. It improves the circulation of oxygen around the body and reduces high blood pressure. It increases the number of red blood cells in your blood plasma; red blood cells carry oxygen. It aids the lymphatic system.

Exercise is modernly known to be so important to mental wellbeing that it is often prescribed by our healthcare system to combat depression. Some research even suggests that exercise is more beneficial in combating depression than anti-depressants.

If you need an instant mood lift, aerobic exercise will most certainly deliver much faster than antidepressants will. This is because when we exercise aerobically, making our hearts and lungs work a little harder than normal, the body secretes chemicals called endorphins. Endorphins are neurotransmitters, those things that aid or inhibit the passage of signals around your nervous system allowing you to experience, feel sensation and move. Endorphins primarily do two things, they block pain receptors, thereby reducing sensation of pain, but they also produce a feeling of euphoria, a 'high' similar to that produced by opiates. They also are thought to be part of the homeostatic process that tells you when you have had enough of a certain thing. So, double whammy there if you are dieting. Exercise does actually make you 'feel' good, as well as being necessary for maintaining the primary body functions such as respiration and circulation.

Anaerobic exercise is a more intense and shorter lasting form of exercise that triggers the fermentation of lactic acid in the muscles. It promotes what we call 'non-endurance' or shorter lasting strength, speed and power and is used by body builders to develop muscle mass. High energy phosphates are stored in small quantities in muscles. These produce energy in the absence of oxygen using glucose or glycogen. The rapid breakdown of glucose results in the formation of lactic acid which is the cause of that muscle burn you feel when anaerobic exercise is performed.

Anaerobic exercise helps to build up endurance, therefore fighting fatigue. It is also thought to help build up the body's ability to eliminate waste and harmful substances.

All forms of exercise should be built up gradually. It is recommended that we build up to at least thirty minutes of aerobic activity every day. This can be very easily built into our everyday lives. Do walk or cycle up to the shop rather than use the car. Do walk slightly faster at times when you are wandering around. Choose to use the stairs rather than the elevator. And do, if you can, introduce a regular workout time into your day, it really does make you feel good as well as benefit your physical wellbeing.

As a nation we tend to pop pills, introducing chemicals into our systems. With a little self-discipline, we wouldn't need to: rather we just look after ourselves.

Start to see yourself in terms of your own worth, your own self value. You are worth looking after, look after yourself and feel happier and healthier in the process. We are made to work perfectly; allow yourself to work perfectly.

Sleep

Lack of sleep makes us feel irritable. Worry and stress can cause lack of sleep. It makes sense then that sleep and feeling good are definitely linked. Furthermore lack of sleep reduces our ability to concentrate. Drive down any motorway and see the signs.

How can we possibly expect to be in control of our own behaviors, (remember actions and reactions), if we do not get enough sleep?

The amount of sleep we need varies between individuals; there is no strictly prescribed amount of sleep you should get. Generally sleep needs are between 6 and 8 hours per night for the average adult. Babies sleep needs can be as great as 17 hours in each 24 hour period.

It is generally accepted there are four stages to our sleep, though some studies use five, splitting the stage 3 section talked of here. We go up and down these stages each night, but not in complete cycles.

Stage 1 is the transitional period between being awake and asleep. During this stage the brain changes from producing alpha waves to very slow theta waves. Lasting approximately 5 to 10 minutes; you feel semi-conscious and may refer to it as drowsing. It is common to experience sudden twitches and jerks in this sleep stage. These are referred to as positive myoclonus. During this stage you begin to lose both muscle tone and conscious awareness of your environment.

Stage 2 is characterized by sleep spindles and K-complexes. Sleep spindles and K-complexes are wave types seen on EEG (electro encephalograms) as a burst of activity and are often followed by muscular twitches. This brain activity has been found to be associated with the integration of new information into existing knowledge, filing in the libraries of our minds so as to speak. This is when knowledge gets stored, relieving the conscious cognitive processes. Cortical arousal is suppressed during this stage, so the brain will not respond to danger stimuli. Consciousness of the external environment disappears completely.

Stage 3 is known as deep sleep or slow wave sleep and is characterised by the production of delta waves. It is during this sleep stage that we are most likely to experience sleepwalking, night terrors or nocturnal enuresis, otherwise known as night time bedwetting.

Stage 4 or REM sleep is characterised by rapid eye movements and higher frequency saw-tooth waves. It is often referred to as paradoxical sleep because whilst the brain becomes more active, muscles experience atonia, a form of paralysis that prevents us from acting out our dreams.

All sleep stages are necessary for optimum physical and mental health. So whilst there is no prescribed time to sleep, it stands to reason that to wake naturally is not going to disturb any of these sleep patterns. It is this we should try to achieve rather than an actual amount of time asleep. Do you have to be woken every day by someone else, or by your alarm clock? Know that you are disturbing sleep cycles if this is the case. You can fix this by allowing yourself to either sleep longer, i.e. until you wake naturally which may be assisted by going to bed earlier.

There are many books and leaflets on sleep hygiene that may be used if sleep problems occur, but the general recommendations are: sleep in an environment that is restful and allocated as your sleeping place, i.e. not the place you do work or play computer games in; try to keep to regular sleeping times; avoid stimulating drinks and foods such as caffeine and cheese just before bedtime; and if you are suffering from stress or anxiety or experiencing worries that keep you awake, use relaxation and/or meditation techniques.

Relaxation and Enjoyment

As well as sleep we need rest. You've heard the old adage - 'a change is as good as a rest' and this is true. Change demands we use different parts of the brain and body; it gives the bits we have been using a chance to rest. Whilst determination and hard effort may be commendable, if we push ourselves too far, it can be counterproductive.

University College London researchers' study of 10,000 English people showed that those who enjoy life the most are three times more likely to live a longer than those who enjoy it the least. Enjoyment is good for your health. What do you enjoy doing? Make sure you spend time doing it.

Also, find enjoyment in everyday things that you do. You have now learned to change your perception. Change your experience of everyday mundane things, shift your perception and look for enjoyment. It is there, see it, feel it. Stop pushing against the inevitable and learn to enjoy things. Fighting against negativity with negativity, increases negativity. Blending negativity with enjoyment and positiveness dilutes the negativity. It is simple math.

Your whole system works well when you are happy. Energy flows, it is its nature. Positive emotions create positive effects throughout your system. Disease is precisely what it says - dis - ease.

The brain particularly works well when you feel relaxed. It is true that many a brilliant business decision was made on the golf course. It is true that many a superb idea was had when sitting there humming. Newton is said to have been relaxing under a tree when he founded the law of gravity!

Relaxation is release of tension, a return to equilibrium. We hold stressors physically in our bodies as well as in our minds. That tense neck and shoulders, the aching jaw from teeth grinding, the thumping headache; these physical pains are signs of tension. Relax.

Sometimes this is easier said than done. If you are not feeling relaxed, use a relaxation technique, one is listed below, but there are many around. Listen to relaxing music. Put your feet up and read a book. Go sit in the sunshine in the garden. Whatever works for you, make sure each and every day you make time to relax; this could be when stuck in a traffic jam! It is important. It will improve the quality of all areas of your life.

Relaxation Technique

Let's take a few minutes to relax your body and mind right now. Ensure you are sitting comfortably and not impeding your circulation in any way; this could be uncrossing your legs or loosening any tight clothing.

We'll begin with a few slow, deep breaths. Each time you breathe in, breathe all the way down into your stomach. Breathe in slowly through your nose, and feel your abdomen and lungs expand with air. Don't rush to breathe in.

After drawing in a long deep breath, allow your breath to flow back out through your mouth. Just let go of each breath, and with it, release any tension or stress you might have been holding on to. You might like to mentally repeat the word "relax" as you breathe out.

Try this now; slowly draw in a deep breath through your nose. Just gradually fill your lungs and abdomen with air, and when they are full, release that breath completely; let your jaw go and allow that air out through your mouth.

You are beginning to feel yourself relaxing. Your breath will dissolve tension just as easily as warm water melts ice.

Breathe in once again. Feel your body fill with air ...and when you are ready, release the breath, let it flow out naturally. Breathe all the way out until your lungs are empty.

Let's draw in a third and final breath, nice and deep. Feel yourself relaxing as you gradually release the breath.

Now let your breathing return to a normal rhythm. Don't rush, take as long as you like.

Become aware of your resting breathing pattern as we begin to scan over your body, looking for areas of tension to release. Let your breath take the rhythm it wants.

As I mention each body part, bring your awareness to it, tense it for a moment and then let it relax. Notice the feeling of relaxation as you do this with each area of your body. Notice how nice it feels as you let go.

It is quite common for people to store a lot of tension in their jaw muscles, so let's begin there. Pay attention to your jaw for a moment. There are a number of very strong muscles in that area. Just momentarily tense as many face muscles as you can, and then – relax. Allow your jaw muscles to loosen and let go. Notice how nice that feels.

Now let your attention wander to the rest of the muscles in your face. Allow your eye muscles to release, and let your cheeks and forehead relax.

Let this peaceful feeling flow slowly down your neck. Feel it sooth your throat and dissolve any tension as it slowly glides down to your shoulders.

Now momentarily tense your shoulders, squeeze them in and up. Now let your shoulders go. Give them a moment of your attention, and just mentally repeat the word "relax" as you let them soften, let go, and release all tension.

Allow that relaxed feeling to spill down your arms.

Now bring your awareness to your arms and tense them momentarily. Then let go. Feel them becoming loose and limp. They are relaxed and at peace, all the way from your shoulders, through your elbows, wrists, right to the tips of your fingers.

Now focus on the muscles in your back...all those muscles surrounding your spine. Tense all those muscles, and those around your tummy and ribcage, and then relax and let go.

Bring your awareness to your chest. Allow your breath to release this area. Imagine your breath whispering to your chest, 'relax'.

As you breathe in and out feel your stomach gently rise and fall. Let your stomach soften and relax with each breath. Feel it releasing tension as each moment passes. You can feel yourself slowly slipping into a state of deep relaxation.

Now bring your attention to your buttocks and thighs, tense them for a moment, then release. Imagine all those strong supporting muscles beginning to relax and unwind. Do the same with your knees ...your calves...your feet. Let them all relax.

Now just enjoy this relaxed feeling for a few moments. It does feel so good.

This relaxed feeling is yours. You have achieved it. Take a mental snapshot of it. Take it with you and bring it to mind throughout your day as you wish to.

Meditation

Relaxation techniques are a helpful introduction to meditation.

Remember Mindful meditation is the mental discipline of directing your attention to your actual experience of this moment. Use breathing as your base. Direct your attention onto your breath; that is the air going in and coming out and the in-between. So notice the air as it commences its journey at the point of your nose. Pay attention to how it feels going down into your lungs. And out through your mouth etcetera.

Whilst you meditate notice how the chair or ground are supporting you. Notice how various parts of your body feel, how various materials feel on your skin. Become aware of all of yourself and your interaction with your environment, smells, and sounds, all of you. Notice how now really feels in all its entirety. In the words of Kabat-Zin, pay attention on purpose to this moment.

As you meditate, you will have thoughts, you will have feelings, you will have physiological responses. Have no expectation of what should or shouldn't occur. Just allow what occurs to occur and observe it. The mental discipline you are learning is to observe in the detached manner of an observer without judgment or prejudice. Observing is passive. You do not need to become involved whatsoever with what you are observing. You are simply observing your own experience.

You can experience and observe at the same time. This is 'awareness'.

So many times I hear 'I can't do it – there's too much noise' or 'something is putting me off'. The point is when you notice the noise or the something, detach yourself, become the observer and observe your own reactions to it. The point of Visapanna meditation is to become aware, non-judgmentally, of your own reactions to things, of your own experience of things.

When you hear a loud noise, a door bangs or someone shouts maybe, you may feel angry, disappointed or let down. You may startle, or you may tense-up. You may find the noise propels your thoughts onto something else. Observe this process in yourself. Where does it start – where does it go? What does it feel like? What emotion did you experience? What happened physiologically – did you tense-up, did your heart begin to beat faster? What words, what head chatter automatically came to mind? These are the things you are observing. Become aware of your own experience – this is the point – this is meditation.

As the observer of yourself, resist the temptation to narrate, to put into words, to judge or to mentally typecast or formulate.

Following your meditation, you do not need to analyse this experience, though of course you will reflect on it. This form of seeing, becoming aware, is TO EXPERIENCE. When it is finished, you have had it, it is done. It is gone as with every experience we have.

What you will find you are left with though is a new knowledge and understanding about yourself. You have created another perspective in which to experience the same experience. You saw how you react, you saw how you felt and to what and where that went. It is this you can use to influence future experiences. You have given yourself another perspective and consequently opened up choice.

By default, this deeper understanding of yourself gives you deeper understanding of others. You do not have to try for this – it simply happens.

You become aware as you realise each second of every day is a new experience in its own right. Everything is seen anew, which is as it really is. Yesterday was not the same as today, tomorrow will be very different. We realise nothing exists in the past or in the future. There is only now – this very moment.

You truly begin to awaken, to live each moment and appreciate that life's richness of experience is always here, now.

This life is as you perceive it, find and choose the perception you want.

Know your own abilities; appreciate what a wonderful job your mind and body do for you. Listen to it.

Acknowledge the hundreds of things you do well. There are so many. Look after you because you are worth looking after.

Judge everything you do by its own merit only. Remember the old saying 'If you judge a fish by its ability to climb walls, it will grow up thinking itself useless'. We do what we do for valid reason. Give yourself a break; acknowledge that.

This moment is yours but only for a moment. In the next moment it has changed.

Bibliography

Anxiety and Depression Association of America. (2010). *Facts & Statistics*. Retrieved March 2nd, 2014, from Anxiety and Depression Association of America: http://www.adaa.org/about-adaa/press-room/facts-statistics

Collins Gem. (2001). *English Dictionary* (New ed.). Glasgow: Harper Collins Publishers Ltd.

Covey, S. R. (2013). *The 7 Habits of Highly Effective People: Powerful Lessons In Personal Change* (25th Anniversary Edition ed.). New York: Simon and Schuster.

Executive, Health and Safety. (2013). *Stress and Psychological Disorders in Great Britain 2013*. United Kingdon: Health and Safety Executive. Retrieved from Health and Safety Executive: http://www.hse.gov.uk/statistics/causdis/stress/

Gunaratana, B. H. (2002). *Mindfulness In Plain English*. Somerville, Canada: Wisdom Publications.

Hicks, E., & Hicks, J. (2007). *The Astonishing Power of Emotions*. London: Hay House UK Ltd.

Kabat-Zin, J. (2013). *Full Catastrophe Living (Revised Edition)*. London: Piatkus, Little Brown Book Company.

Marieb, E. N. (2009). *Essentials of Human Anatomy & Physiology* (Ninth ed.). San Fransisco, USA: Pearson Benjamin Cummings.

Maxwell, G., Finch, S. (Producers), & Maxwell, G. (Director). (2010). *Invisible Worlds* [Motion Picture]. Retrieved March 6th, 2014, from http://www.bbc.co.uk/programmes/b00rmrmm/clips

National Institute for Health and Clinical Excellence. (2011). *Welcome to the National Institute for Health and Clinical Excellence.*

(National Institute for Health and Clinical Excellence)
Retrieved November 23rd, 2011, from National Institute for
Health and Clinical Excellence: http://www.nice.org.uk/

Nicholson, A. (2013). *Oh Why Did I Do That!? ... and what to do about it.* London: Esteem World Publications.

Page, R. (2002). *The Enlightened Response.* Chichester: Nutshell.

Perlmutter FACN, D. D., & Villoldo PhD, A. (2011). *Power Up Your Brain.* London: Hay House UK Ltd.

Sainsbury Centre for Mental Health. (2008). Ten Top Tips for Recovery Orientated Practice. London: Sainsbury Centre for Mental Health.

Thomas, B., & Harding, S. &. (1997). *Mental Health Nursing Principles and Practice.*

Wachowski, A., & Wachowski, L. (Directors). (1999). *The Matrix* [Motion Picture].

Williams, H. (2009, November 10). Foods to beat depression. *The Independant.*

Winston, R. (2002). *Human Instinct.* London: Transworld Pulbishers.

Winston, R. (2003). *The Human Mind: And how to make the most of it.* London: Bantam Press.

Reviews – Oh Why Did I Do That!? ... and what to do about it Copyright © 2013 Amanda Nicholson

In Mandy Nicholson's 'Oh why did I do that!?...and what to do about it' key elements of developmental and behavioural psychology, neurophysiology and linguistics are interwoven from an informed first person perspective to present mindfulness in a readily understandable and practicable format. Mandy is a naturally confident narrator who writes with motivation and an immediacy and clarity that both fascinates and informs as it inspires. This book is designed to help you develop a more positive and successful attitude towards yourself and your life by rethinking what does and doesn't work for you in the mindfulness context of acknowledgement and acceptance. The author has the self-insight, emotional intelligence and literary skill to make this a self-help book that does what it says; helps you to help yourself. This is definitely a book that I will benefit from rereading again and again.

Dr Sarah Markham

It's about options – and enables the reader to choose the options that help them help themselves – simple, easy to read and a gem of a book

Bev Blanchard

This book tells you a lot about yourself! I usually struggle with 'self-help' books, but this one gave plenty of insight into why we do things and gives tips and help in avoiding similar things happening in the future, without being 'too deep' and (for me) boring. I read the whole book in one evening and would certainly recommend it to a friend.

TJ Clark "Aviation Historian"

Real Life Mindful Practices for a Calm and Less Stressed Life!,

The author knows what she is talking about. This explains mindfulness and how it can be brought into everyday life. It is something we all can do – something that can change our reactions and beliefs.

Phillip Levine (Norwalk, CT USA)

I'm fairly new to working in a mental health setting and wanted a book to tell me about mindfulness in a hurry to get up to speed quickly. This book does that. It's like sitting down with the author whiles she says, this is what it is... It provides a grounding in mindfulness and enabled me to move on to Jon Kabat-Zin's book with confidence.

Liz Tremlett – Senior Occupational Therapist

www.ingramcontent.com/pod-product-compliance
Lightning Source LLC
Chambersburg PA
CBHW051713170526
45167CB00002B/640